GORDON RAMSAY'S ULTIMATE FIT FOOD

GORDON RAMSAY'S ULTIMATE FIT FOOD

HODDER &
STOUGHTON

First published in Great Britain in 2018
by Hodder & Stoughton
An Hachette UK company

1

Copyright © Gordon Ramsay 2018

Photography copyright © Jamie Orlando Smith 2018

A CIP catalogue record for this title is available from
the British Library

Hardback ISBN 978 1 473 65227 9
Ebook ISBN 978 1 473 65228 6

Colour origination by Born Group
Printed and bound in Germany by Mohn Media

Hodder & Stoughton policy is to use papers that are
natural, renewable and recyclable products and made
from wood grown in sustainable forests. The logging and
manufacturing processes are expected to conform to the
environmental regulations of the country of origin.

Editorial Director: Nicky Ross
Project Editor: Natalie Bradley
Editor: Camilla Stoddart
Nutritionist: Kerry Torrens
Copy-editor: Annie Lee
Designer & Art Director: James Edgar
Photographer: Jamie Orlando Smith
Food Stylist: Phil Mundy
Props Stylist: Olivia Wardle
Shoot Producer: Ruth Ferrier
Art Director: Alasdair Oliver
Production Manager: Claudette Morris

Hodder & Stoughton Ltd
Carmelite House
50 Victoria Embankment
London EC4Y 0DZ

www.hodder.co.uk

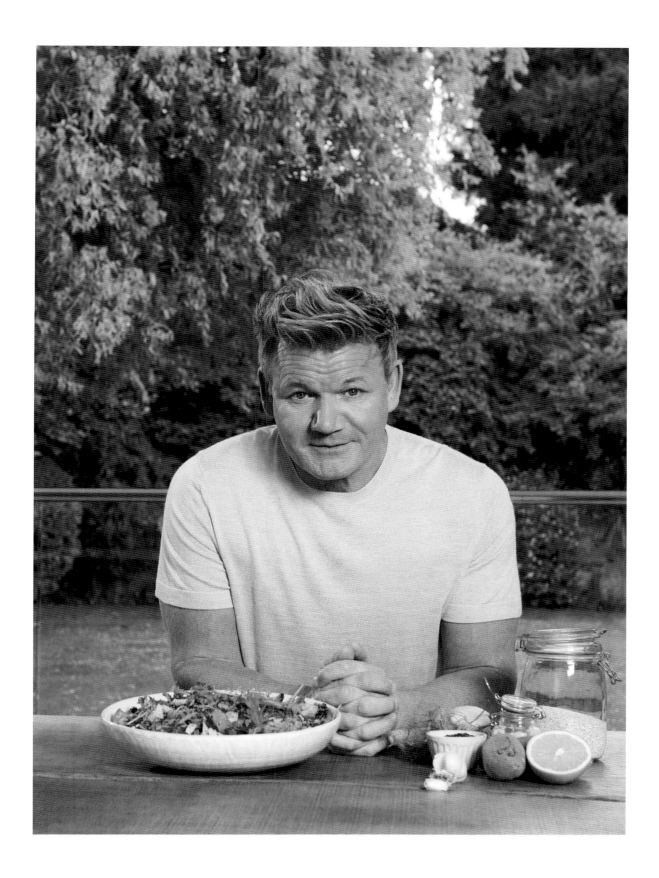

CONTENTS

CONTENTS

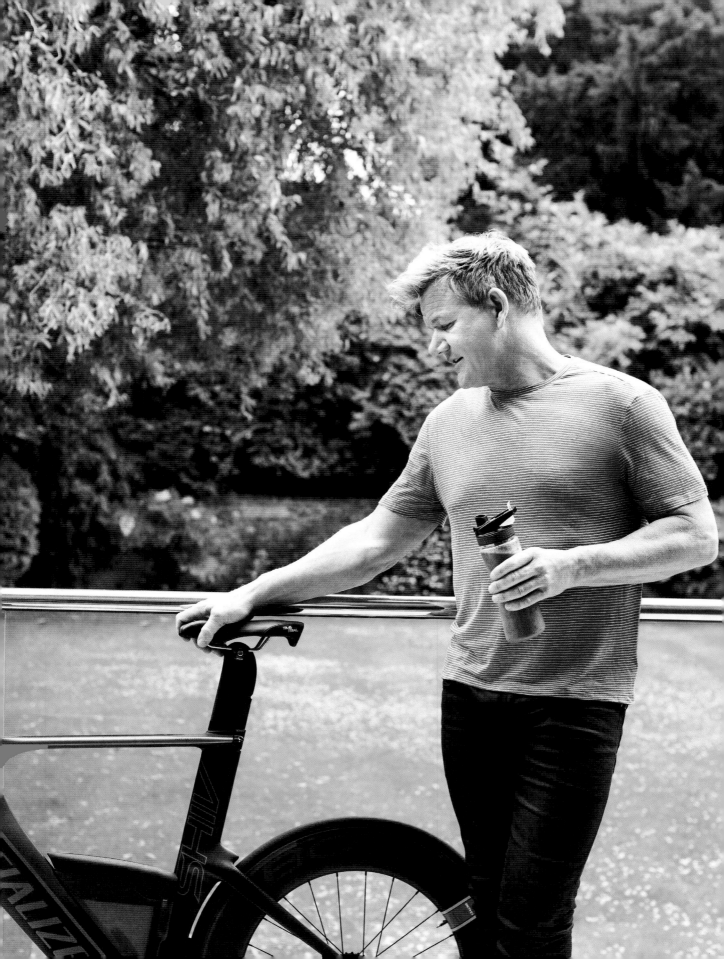

INTRODUCTION

I HAVE ALWAYS SAID THAT CHEFS EAT THE BEST FOOD AND THE WORST IN EQUAL MEASURE.

They work with the freshest, most delicious ingredients available, cook them perfectly and are constantly trying little tasty mouthfuls as they work. But do they get home and make themselves a nutritious meal at the end of their 16-hour shift? I'm afraid they do not. The punishing working life of a chef means that they often rely on junk food and sugary snacks to get through the day, and finding time for exercise is really hard. When I was working in the restaurant at Royal Hospital Road, I never left the kitchen, sending everyone else out on their break rather than getting out myself, and I was snacking on the wrong things throughout the day. Over time, I let myself get out of shape. My chef's whites got tighter and tighter and I felt lethargic and sluggish a lot of the time.

It all changed when I started forcing myself to go to the gym for a run. I had to schedule it in like a trip to the dentist so I couldn't get out of it! I started with 5km, then 10km, then, before I knew it, I was running my first marathon! That was followed later the same year with an ultramarathon in South Africa ... I was hooked. Being fit made me feel great and it became my escape from my very busy life. My eating improved, the weight came off and I looked and felt so much better. My health improved dramatically, too. I turned 50 recently and, given that my father died of a heart attack at 53, Tana organized a complete health check-up for me. I was in training for the Ironman Triathlon World Championship in Hawaii at the time and when they checked my pulse, it was the lowest resting heart rate for a man of my age that they had ever seen! I must be doing something right ...

For me, being healthy involves eating well and taking exercise. This sounds obvious but I can't stress enough the importance of doing these things in combination (though not necessarily at the same time!). To improve your diet without exercising can only get you so far when you are trying to lose weight or boost your health. Similarly, to take up exercising without considering what you eat will have only limited success. It is the combination of the two that brings better health.

But this is not a diet book telling you what (and what not) to eat, nor is it full of faddy ideas about eating cabbage soup or living off grapefruits or eating like a caveman. It works on the very simple premise that what you put into your body makes a difference to how it functions. It also acknowledges that the body has different requirements depending on what you are expecting it to do. If you are trying to lose a bit of weight you need to eat less than when you are maintaining a healthy weight, and when you are taking part in rigorous exercise you will need to fuel your body correctly to ensure it has the resources to deliver.

Finally, healthy eating doesn't have to be dull! As a chef, I want the food that I eat to be tasty and satisfying as well as good for me. When I'm in training, I don't want my taste buds to get bored by eating the same things over and over again. And I don't ever want to feel deprived. These are my go-to recipes when I want to eat well at home, and my great hope is that they will inspire you to get cooking to improve your own health whatever your personal goal. Here's to better health!

Gordan x

WHAT IS HEALTHY EATING?

I am not going to get scientific here, but I do think an understanding of what the body needs and how it gets this from food can help us make better decisions when it comes to eating. I am lucky enough to have worked with personal trainers and nutritionists who have shared their knowledge with me and, once I learnt the basics, making healthy decisions has become second nature.

To keep itself properly fuelled and in optimum condition, the body needs a combination of macro- and micronutrients. Macronutrients are foods we need in relatively large amounts. The main three are:

PROTEIN – found in meat, fish, dairy produce, eggs, pulses, beans and nuts, and essential for building and repairing tissue in bones, muscles, cartilage, skin and blood as well as for the production of hormones and important enzymes. The recommended daily intake for protein is 50g for women and 55g for men.

CARBOHYDRATES – the starches, sugars and dietary fibre found in foods such as potatoes, grains (like wheat, rice, corn, etc.), pulses, fruit and vegetables which are the body's main source of energy. Fibre found in starchy carbohydrates is essential for digestive health; it helps with the elimination of waste and can prevent heart disease, some cancers and diabetes. The recommended daily intake for carbohydrates is 260g for women and 300g for men, and health experts recommend a daily intake of roughly 30g of fibre for both men and women.

FAT – an excellent source of energy and needed for the absorption of some vital micronutrients. Confusingly, all fats are not created equal, so while the body does need some fat to survive, it is healthy unsaturated fat and not saturated fat that is required (see page 25 for more information). Fat is found in oils, animal products, fish, seeds and nuts. The recommended daily intake of fat should be limited to 70g for women and 95g for men, of which no more than 20g and 30g respectively should be saturated fat.

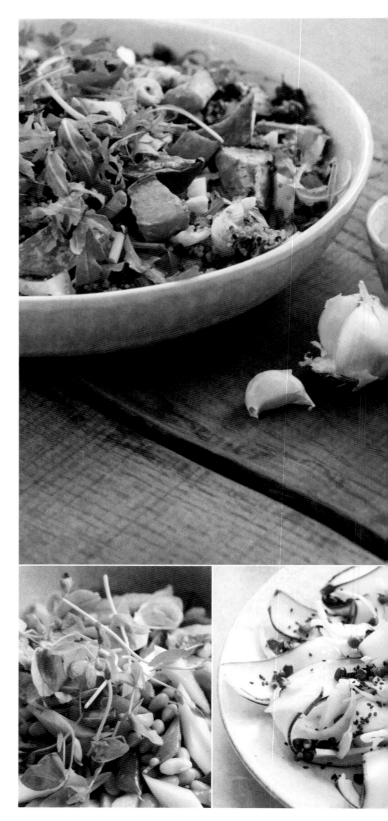

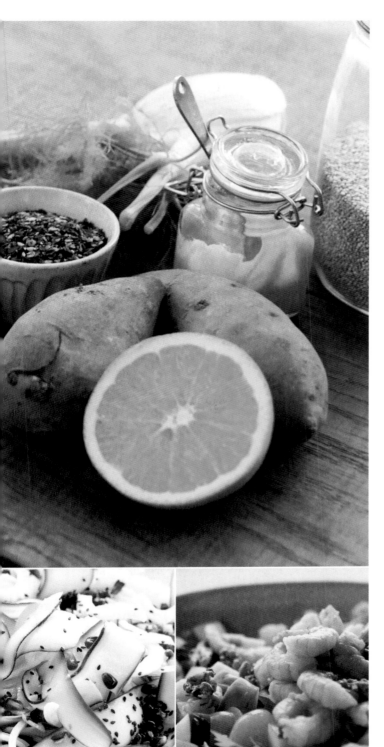

Micronutrients are the vitamins and minerals that we need in much smaller amounts but that are no less vital for normal growth and healthy development. Micronutrients include vitamins A, B complex (including folic acid), C, D, E and K as well as minerals like iron, calcium, magnesium, potassium and zinc. Vitamins and minerals are found in lots of different foods, including vegetables, fruit, nuts, eggs and dairy produce, and they are important for the smooth running of our organs, eyes, skin, gut, immune system, etc. No one food or meal contains all the vitamins and minerals we need, which is why eating a varied diet is so important.

Everything the body needs is available from the food we eat so we should all be pretty healthy, right? Unfortunately it isn't quite as simple as that. The problem is that there are some things that we don't need a lot of, like refined carbohydrates, saturated fat and sugar (see page 24), but we eat lots of them because they taste good – think crisps, fizzy drinks, fast food, cakes and biscuits. Not only can these things be detrimental to our health when eaten in excess, if we regularly choose to fill ourselves up with the bad stuff, we are likely to be consuming too many calories and missing out on the vital nutrients and fibre present in healthier foods.

The body's requirements change if you are trying to lose weight (see page 109) and also if you lead a very active lifestyle (see page 189), but generally we should all be trying to eat as varied a diet as possible while keeping our intake of saturated fat, sugar and salt down (see page 23). The recipes in this book will make it easy to eat the right variety of foods depending on the challenges you face.

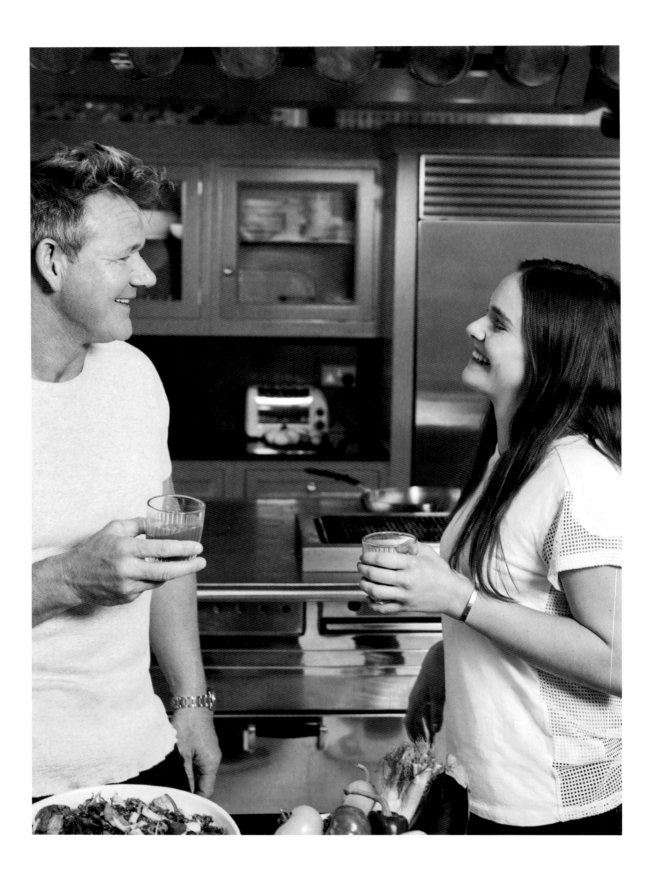

HEALTHY KIDS

It is especially important that children get all the macro- and micronutrients that they need while they are growing and developing. The exact nutritional requirements of children and teenagers are beyond the remit of this book, but I do think that introducing kids to a wide variety of foods including plenty of fruit and vegetables from a young age helps them to develop a taste for healthy foods, and by keeping fried, processed fatty, salty and overly sweet foods to a minimum, you can teach them that these are treats to be indulged in only once in a while. Making smoothies, soups and veg-packed stews and sauces is an excellent way to pack as many nutrients as possible into growing kids, even the most veg-avoiding ones, and eating together as a family can encourage your children to try new things when they see what the adults are eating.

But to me, it isn't just a case of what you feed children; it's about teaching them to make good choices and equipping them with the skills they need to look after themselves when they leave your care, skills like basic nutrition and cooking. Ever since our four children were tiny, it has been important to Tana and me that they have a good understanding of food – where it comes from, how to cook it and how it affects our health. They are now teenagers and it seems to have paid off. Sure they all like pizza, chocolate and fizzy drinks like everyone else, but most of the time they eat a healthy, varied diet that balances out the special treats. They also understand the important relationship between diet and exercise and are really active. I like to think we have given them a really healthy relationship with food for life.

There are lots of family-friendly recipes in this book but it should be noted that children should not follow a low-fat diet unless instructed to by a doctor. Healthy fats are particularly vital for children's development, so restricting fat is not recommended.

HOW TO USE
THIS BOOK

Each of the dishes in this book has been analysed by a nutritionist and the figures are printed alongside each recipe to help you to become familiar with the nutritional content of everyday meals. These figures exclude optional items and garnishes. Based on these numbers, I have split the recipes into three sections – Healthy, Lean and Fit.

There are no rigid rules, though. You can mix and match recipes from the different sections depending on who you are cooking for. For example, you can add a Healthy side dish to a Lean main course if you are feeding children and non-dieters, or you can serve a carbohydrate-boosting side dish from the Fit section with a healthy supper if you are in training for a race or event. Just keep an eye on the figures over the course of a day to check you aren't taking in more calories than you actually need.

Here are the official Reference Intake (RI) guidelines for moderately active men and women. These indicate what you need in a day for a healthy, balanced diet. Keep these in mind when you are planning your meals to make sure you are adequately fuelling your day. You should aim not to exceed the figures listed below for fat, saturated fat, sugar and salt. Individual needs may vary, so this should be used as a guide only.

	WOMEN	MEN
KCAL	2,000	2,500
FAT (G)	70	95
SATURATES (G)	20	30
CARBS (G)	260	300
SUGARS (G)	90	120
PROTEIN (G)	50	55
SALT (G)	6	6

HEALTHY

To be categorized as Healthy, one serving has to contain:

— no more than 5g of saturated fat
— no more than 15g of sugar
— no more than 1.5g of salt per serving

These recipes are ideal for maintaining a healthy weight, keeping blood sugar levels stable and boosting your intake of a wide variety of nutrients.

LEAN

The dishes in the Lean section come in at:

— under 300 calories per serving for breakfast
— under 600 calories per serving for lunch and dinner
— under 150 calories for a snack

Also, a limited number of the calories are derived from fat. Choosing recipes from this section will help you to consume fewer calories, which in turn will help you to lose weight over a period of time, especially when combined with raised activity levels.

FIT

The Fit section is full of meals and snacks that contain the right amounts, types and combinations of macronutrients (carbohydrate, protein and fat) for an active lifestyle. These recipes provide:

— fuel for training and endurance sports
— proteins for recovery and repairing tired muscles

There are more calories in some of these dishes to meet the needs of the body when exercising.

NOTES ABOUT
THE INGREDIENTS

ANIMAL WELFARE

Try to buy meat, eggs and dairy products from reputable farms that value the welfare of their livestock. It isn't just better for the animals, it is better for you, as it is likely to be a more flavourful product.

LOW-FAT FOODS

At home, we try to eat ingredients in their most natural form so we can be sure of what we are putting into our bodies. Avoid low-fat versions of favourites because they often contain lots of sugar to make up for the lack of flavour. That said, low-fat dairy products like semi-skimmed milk, reduced fat coconut milk and 0% fat Greek yoghurt make it into this book when keeping fat levels down is important.

ORGANIC INGREDIENTS

Choose organic ingredients where you can as they contain lower levels of pesticides and heavy metals and more nutrients. They have less impact on the environment, too, so it's a win–win.

EGGS

All eggs in this book are medium-sized unless otherwise stated. Always buy free-range eggs if you can.

FISH

Choose fish from sustainable sources, caught or farmed using environmentally friendly methods.

OIL

In this book, I mostly use olive, rapeseed and groundnut oils for frying and extra virgin olive oil for dressing, drizzling and finishing. When choosing coconut oil, make sure it is the unrefined 'virgin' variety which is rich in a useful form of saturated fats (see page 25 for more information about coconut oil).

HERBS

A small bunch of herbs weighs 25–30g and a large bunch weighs 50–60g.

SALT

I season my food with sea salt because it enhances the flavour but you can leave it out if you are trying to keep your salt levels down.

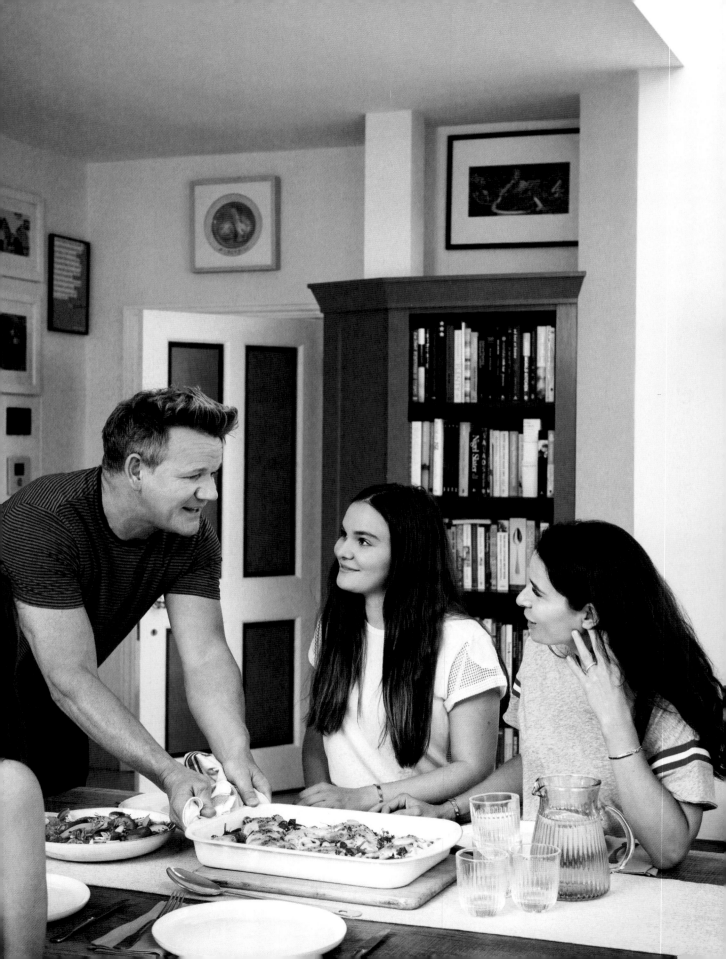

NOURISHING
BREAKFASTS

NUTRITIOUS LUNCHES
AND SALADS

SUPER SUPPERS
AND SIDES

HEALTHY SNACKS AND
NOT-TOO-SWEET TREATS

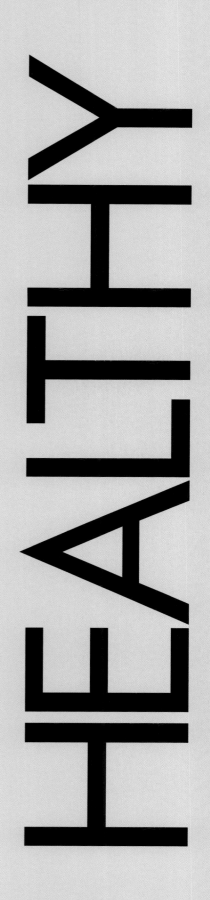

HEALTHY

THERE IS A LOT OF MISINFORMATION ABOUT HEALTHY EATING AROUND THESE DAYS.

It is widely agreed that consuming a diet of fried chicken, chips, cake and biscuits is not balanced or likely to be very beneficial for health! Our usual response is to try to cut down on the bad things like sugar, fat and salt to improve our wellbeing. But to me, healthy eating is not just about avoiding the foods that we know are bad for us but about actively seeking out the good things and trying to eat as varied a diet as possible. This chapter is all about making good choices and finding new ways to add healthy ingredients to your meals.

One of the best ways to increase the amount and variety of nutrients and fibre in your diet is to consume more fruit and vegetables. The UK government recommends aiming to eat at least five portions every day, but recent findings suggest this number should be even higher. Happily, I love most fruit and veg, but I still need inspiration when it comes to trying new ones or finding ways to increase my daily intake. The salads, side dishes, soups and even the snacks in this section will make hitting your five-a-day really easy.

Another way to eat your way towards better health is to ensure that you include lots of so-called superfoods in your diet. This term is controversial, because there is no official definition of a superfood, but it is generally considered to be an ingredient that punches above its weight in nutritional terms. The list includes nutrient-rich giants such as broccoli, avocado, kale, spinach, blueberries, quinoa, eggs, walnuts and oily fish. While none of these foods have any actual magic powers, a diet that features a variety of superfoods will be very nutritious and a really positive step in the right direction.

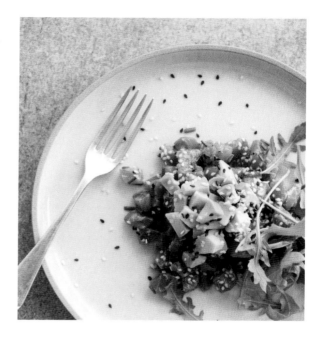

As well as eating more beneficial foods, a great way to instantly improve your health is to cook more yourself. Many people rely on the quick fix of ready meals without realizing that they are often very high in fat, salt and sugar, not to mention artificial colours, flavourings, emulsifiers and stabilizers, etc. In restaurant kitchens, almost everything is made from scratch, so the food, however fancy, is actually very simple. If you cook from scratch at home, you will always know exactly what goes into your meals (and into your mouth) and you can keep the all-important fat, salt and sugar levels down.

The great bonus of improving the quality of the food you eat is that over time you will crave the bad stuff less and less. Your tastes will start to change and you find healthy meals and snacks more satisfying than the greasy, sugary quick fixes you used to eat without thinking. It's a virtuous circle – the better the food you eat, the better you feel, and the better you feel, the better food choices you make, the ultimate winner being your long-term health. You just have to get started . . .

REFINED CARBOHYDRATES AND SUGAR

When you begin to learn about nutrition, you discover that it isn't always straightforward. Take carbohydrates, for example; all carbs provide the body with energy, but it turns out that there are good and bad sources. So-called 'good' carbs are also known as complex carbohydrates because they are relatively difficult for the body to digest, due to their chemical structure and their fibre content. They tend to be whole or unrefined and because they take longer to break down, the energy they provide is released slowly and steadily for the body to access over time. Good sources of complex carbs include wholemeal bread, brown pasta, jumbo oats, brown rice, peas, beans and starchy vegetables. These carbs also provide a wide range of vitamins and minerals and will make you feel fuller for longer, thanks to the dietary fibre.

'Bad' carbs, on the other hand, are known as simple carbs and are either naturally very easy to digest (e.g. sugar) or have been processed or cooked in a way that removes all the good stuff that usually slows down digestion. These refined carbs are found in white bread, white pasta, biscuits, cakes and baked goods made with white flour. The lack of dietary fibre in these foods means that the energy they provide hits the bloodstream really quickly, causing blood sugar levels to spike and crash and leaving you tired, irritable, light-headed and hungry for more. Over time, these fluctuating sugar levels may lead to weight gain, which can increase your risk of developing health problems like heart disease and possibly diabetes.

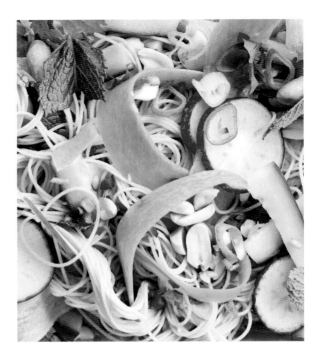

Because nutrition isn't straightforward, there are two types of sugar, too. Naturally occurring sugars are found in fruit, vegetables and dairy products and are not considered a problem for health as long as they are eaten in the form that nature intended; in fact, they can be an excellent source of accessible energy. But the other type, known as 'free' sugar, is definitely considered a problem. Free sugars include those that are added to our food, like regular sugar, white and brown, as well as other sweeteners such as honey, maple syrup, corn syrup, palm sugar, agave syrup and fruit juices. It is these sugars that we are advised to cut down on, because they provide lots of calories without much or any goodness and we tend to consume too much of them, not least because they are often hidden in ready meals, snacks and fizzy drinks to make them taste better. Consuming too much sugar is one of the major causes of obesity and tooth decay around the world, and cutting back is a really positive way to improve your health. The recipes in this book do include free sugars such as honey, maple syrup and agave syrup, but in small quantities and combined with complex carbohydrates and sometimes protein to slow down their effect.

FAT

Fat has had a hard time over the years. It's been blamed for obesity, raised cholesterol levels and heart disease, and we have been told to keep our intake to a minimum. But like many pieces of nutritional advice, the reality is not so simple; it turns out we actually need some fat in our diet to stay healthy. It's a valuable source of energy and is essential for the absorption of various important vitamins like A, D, E and K and for the production of hormones.

Like sugar and carbs, there are two main types of fat and, historically, saturated fat found in animal products like lard, butter and cheese has been considered 'bad' fat, while unsaturated fats from plant sources like olive, sunflower and nut oils, as well as oily fish, is thought of as 'good' fat. But a number of recent studies are questioning these long-held beliefs and are suggesting that saturated fat isn't quite as bad for us as previously thought. While this may be good news for those of us who enjoy a nicely marbled steak and cooking with butter from time to time, the government guidelines haven't changed and we are still advised to keep our intake of saturated fat to below 20g a day for women and 30g for men.

Some of the recipes in this book use coconut oil, which is worth mentioning here because although it comes from a plant, it actually contains a lot of saturated fat – but it's a special type of saturated fat which is thought to be helpful for weight loss by both reducing appetite and boosting metabolism. When buying coconut oil, choose the unrefined virgin variety because it is rich in these special fats.

There are also other forms of fat which are critical to good health; these essential fats (known as omega-3) are good for your heart and important for learning and behaviour. Good sources include oily fish like salmon and trout and, to a lesser extent, nuts and seeds like walnuts, chia and flaxseeds, and we should actively try to consume more of them.

Whether the fat comes from saturated or unsaturated sources, the key thing to remember is that fat provides, gram for gram, over twice as much energy as carbohydrates and protein. So if you are consuming too much fat without burning it off through exercise, the excess energy will be stored as body fat. Whatever recent findings about fat being good for you, it is no time to celebrate with a plate of fish and chips!

A WORD ABOUT HYDRATION

Almost more important than what you eat is how much you drink … A human being can survive more than three weeks without eating but would die after three days without water. At least 60% of the body is water and it is vital to keep liquid levels topped up throughout the day, particularly if you are taking exercise (see page 191 for more information about hydrating for sport). It is recommended that we drink 6–8 glasses of water a day to ward off dehydration, which can give you a headache and make you feel irritable and drowsy. Happily, other drinks such as coffee, tea, milk, fruit juice and smoothies all count towards your liquid intake over the day. On top of this, about 20% of the fluid we consume comes from the food that we eat, especially if we eat lots of fruit and vegetables – another reason to aim to beat our five-a-day target.

NOURISHING BREAKFASTS

APPLE, MINT, SPINACH, LIME AND CUCUMBER JUICE

SERVES 2

A freshly squeezed juice is a great, vitamin-packed way to start the day. It wakes up the taste buds and rehydrates the body after a long night's sleep. Juices count as one of your five-a-day so you'll be getting off to a racing start before you have even eaten your breakfast. This is particularly good for getting kids to eat spinach because they won't be able to taste it. You could also serve it on ice as a really refreshing mocktail for summer entertaining.

1 green apple, cored and quartered
4 mint sprigs, leaves only
2 big handfuls of spinach leaves, washed
Juice of 1½ limes
½ cucumber, roughly chopped

1. Put all the ingredients into a juicer or blender and blend until smooth. If the mixture needs a little help going through a juicer then add a little cold water as you juice.

2. Serve in a tall glass with ice.

PER SERVING	
KCAL	48
FAT (g)	1.0
SATURATES (g)	0.1
CARBS (g)	7.0
SUGARS (g)	7.0
FIBRE (g)	1.0
PROTEIN (g)	2.0
SALT (g)	0.03

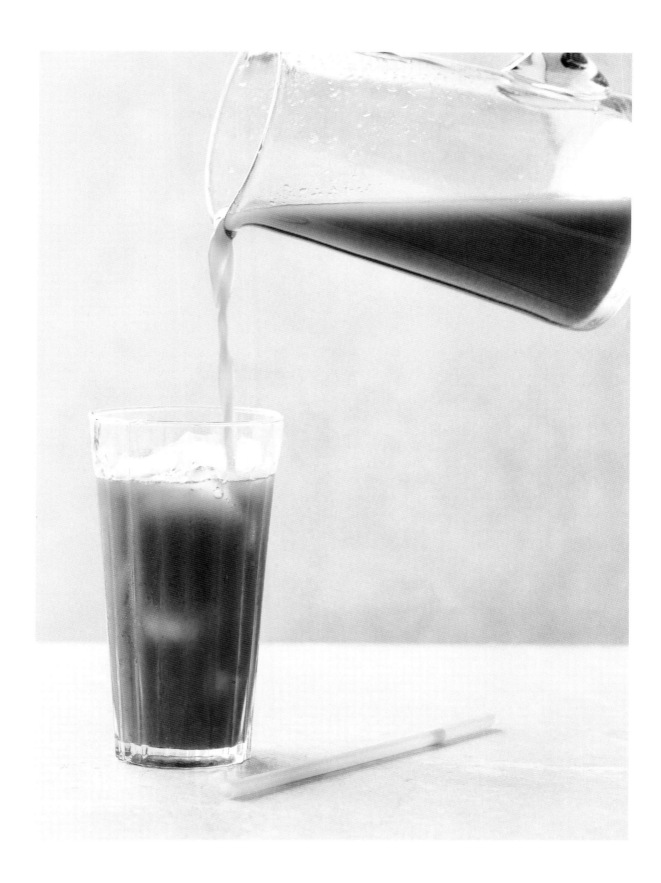

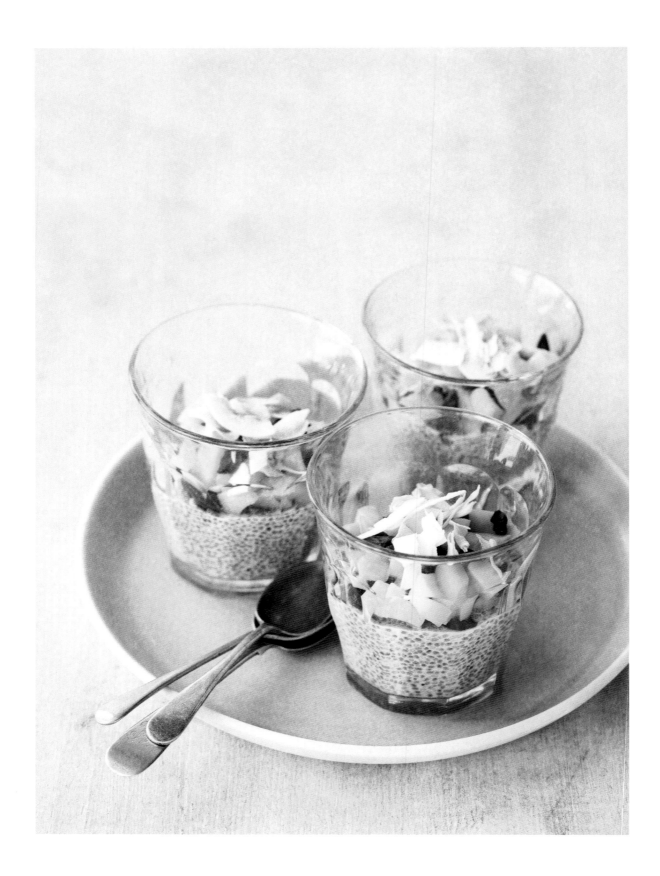

TROPICAL CHIA SEED PUDDING

SERVES 4

My wife Tana introduced me to this very fashionable, light breakfast. She's a really healthy eater and gets the rest of us to eat our greens and try new things like chia seeds, coconut water and goji berries. Chia seeds are full of good things like plant proteins, fibre, antioxidants, omega-3 fatty acids and minerals, but they're not just really good for you, they're also really clever – they can absorb approximately ten times their own weight in liquid, which is how they are magically turned into these delicious breakfast bowls.

320ml coconut milk drink
80g chia seeds
½ tsp vanilla extract
1 mango, diced
2 tbsp goji berries
2 tbsp toasted coconut flakes (optional)

1. Pour the coconut milk into a measuring jug.

2. Divide the chia seeds between four breakfast bowls and add approximately 80ml of the coconut liquid and a drop of vanilla extract to each bowl.

3. Cover and place in the fridge for at least 1 hour, or overnight.

4. Once ready to eat, put the diced mango and goji berries on top of the chia seeds and sprinkle over the toasted coconut, if using.

VARIATIONS

Chia seed pudding can also be made with other milks, such as almond, rice, soya, oat or cow's, and topped with different fruits, nuts and seeds, so experiment with flavours that you like – just remember the basic ratio of one part chia seeds to four parts liquid.

PER SERVING	
KCAL	160
FAT (g)	8.0
SATURATES (g)	2.0
CARBS (g)	13.0
SUGARS (g)	10.0
FIBRE (g)	9.0
PROTEIN (g)	5.0
SALT (g)	0.20

RASPBERRY CHIA SEED JAM

MAKES 1 X 340G JAR

This is the quickest, easiest and healthiest jam recipe around. It uses the gelling power of chia seeds to transform a couple of punnets of raspberries into jam without having to worry about special pans, thermometers, pectin, etc. And it's good for you too! The amount of honey will depend on the ripeness of the raspberries, so taste as you go.

250g fresh raspberries (see below)
Juice of ½ lemon
2–3 tbsp runny honey, to taste
3 tbsp chia seeds

1. Put the raspberries and lemon juice into a blender with 2 tbsp of honey and blitz until smooth. Taste and add a little more honey if necessary.

2. Add the chia seeds and briefly blitz again to mix.

3. Transfer to a clean 340g jar with a lid and allow to set in the fridge for 1 hour. This will keep for a few days in the fridge.

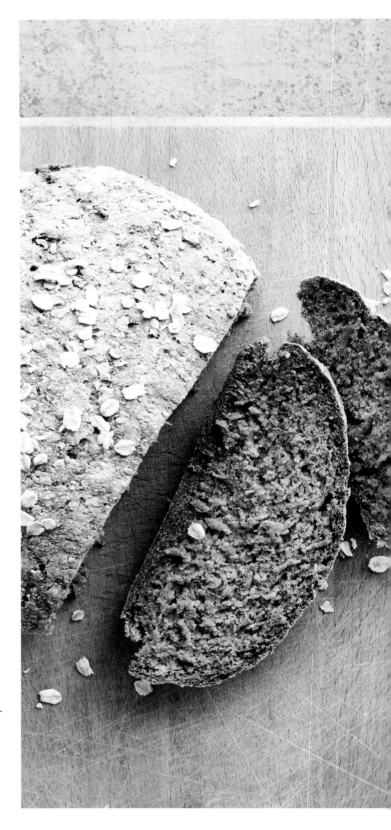

PER TABLESPOON	
KCAL	17
FAT (g)	1.0
SATURATES (g)	0.1
CARBS (g)	1.0
SUGARS (g)	1.0
FIBRE (g)	1.0
PROTEIN (g)	0.5
SALT (g)	0.0

VARIATION
You can also use frozen raspberries for this recipe which means you can make delicious jam all year round. Defrost the fruit slightly before blitzing.

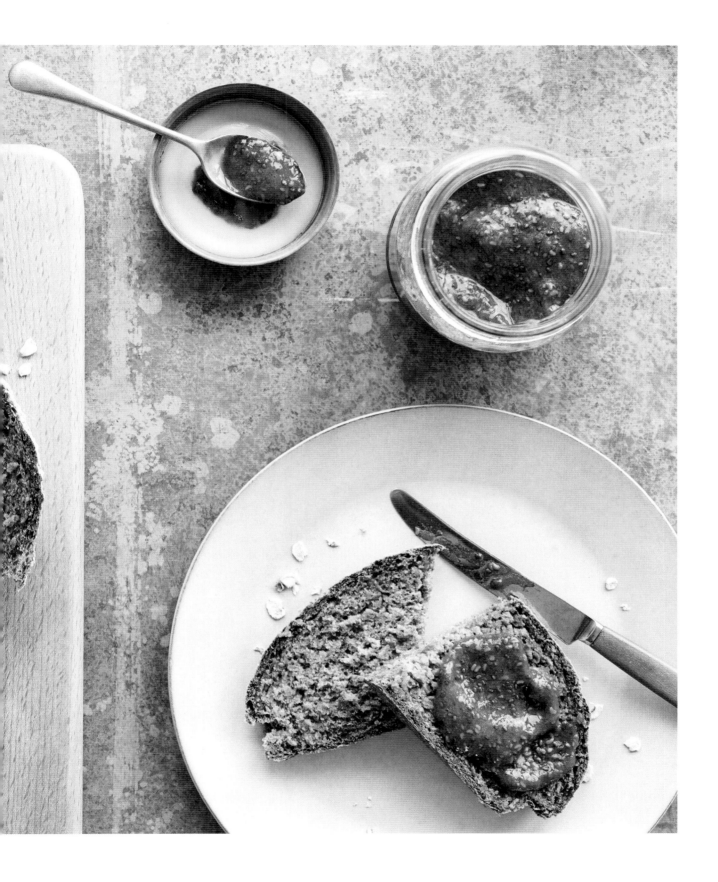

TOASTED OAT SODA BREAD

MAKES 1 LARGE LOAF (ROUGHLY 12 SLICES)

If you have never baked bread before, a traditional Irish soda bread is a really good place to start. It is 'raised' with bicarbonate of soda rather than yeast, so there is no need to wait around for it to prove, and it's pretty difficult for it to go wrong. Toasting the oats before adding them gives them a darker colour and nutty flavour that works really well here. It is especially delicious toasted and served with the Raspberry Chia Seed Jam on page 32.

Flavourless oil, e.g. groundnut, for greasing
125g rolled oats, plus extra for scattering
  over the surface
275ml boiling water
200ml buttermilk, plus a little extra for brushing
  (see below)
150ml skimmed milk
2 tsp bicarbonate of soda
400g wholemeal flour
1 tsp fine salt

1. Preheat the oven to 200°C/gas 6. Grease a 23cm non-stick cake tin with a little oil.

2. Scatter the oats over a baking tray and place in the oven for 30 minutes, turning occasionally. The oats should become nutty and dark in colour.

3. Tip the browned oats straight into a large bowl and pour over the boiling water. Leave the oats to soak until the water has cooled completely.

4. Reduce the oven temperature to 180°C/gas 4.

5. Add the buttermilk and milk to the oats and water, then beat until thoroughly incorporated. Beat in the bicarbonate of soda, flour and salt until fully mixed.

6. Tip the mixture into the cake tin and bake in the preheated oven for 20 minutes. Quickly remove from the oven, brush with a little buttermilk, then scatter over a small handful of oats and return to the oven for a further 30 minutes. If the bread is colouring too much, cover with tin foil for the remaining time.

7. Leave the bread to cool completely in the tin, then, when cool enough to handle, tip it out and serve.

PER SLICE	
KCAL	171
FAT (g)	2.0
SATURATES (g)	0.3
CARBS (g)	31.0
SUGARS (g)	2.0
FIBRE (g)	4.0
PROTEIN (g)	6.0
SALT (g)	0.90

VARIATION
If you can't buy buttermilk, use ordinary milk instead, but add a level teaspoon of cream of tartar with the bicarbonate of soda.

OAT AND QUINOA PORRIDGE WITH MIXED SEEDS

SERVES 4

Being Scottish, I eat porridge for breakfast all the time. I must know over a hundred different ways of serving it! This version has added quinoa, which gives it a bit of crunch as well as being a source of complete protein, extra fibre and energizing B vitamins. Topping it off with berries and mixed seeds makes it the healthiest porridge I know.

175g quinoa, rinsed
75g jumbo rolled oats
200g fresh berries, e.g. raspberries,
    blackberries, strawberries and blueberries
4 tbsp mixed seeds, e.g. sunflower,
    pumpkin and linseeds
Maple syrup, to taste
Sea salt

1. Bring 1 litre of water and a pinch of salt to a simmer in a heavy-based saucepan. Once simmering, stir in the quinoa and cook gently for 10 minutes, stirring occasionally.

2. Add the oats and stir. Continue to simmer for a further 10 minutes, or until thick and porridge-like.

3. Remove the pan from the heat and divide the porridge between serving bowls. Top with the berries, sprinkle over the seeds and drizzle with a little maple syrup for extra sweetness. Serve immediately.

HOW TO MAKE AHEAD
To speed things up in the morning, pre-cook the quinoa and soak overnight with the oats, so all you need to do is heat it through the next morning. Just reduce the amount of liquid you use to cook the porridge by 200ml.

PER SERVING	
KCAL	315
FAT (g)	10.0
SATURATES (g)	1.0
CARBS (g)	40.0
SUGARS (g)	5.0
FIBRE (g)	8.0
PROTEIN (g)	12.0
SALT (g)	0.20

APPLE-PIE-SPICED PORRIDGE

SERVES 4

This is another of my favourite porridge recipes, this time flavoured with apple-pie spices and sweetened with apples and dates, which goes down really well with the junior members of my family – it tastes like pudding! It's especially warming and delicious and the perfect thing to get you out of bed on a cold winter's morning. And with its slow-releasing energy, it should keep you going until lunchtime.

150g jumbo rolled oats
4 dates, stoned and finely chopped
½ tsp ground cinnamon
Pinch of freshly grated nutmeg
Pinch of ground allspice
2 eating apples, cored and cut into chunks
400ml semi-skimmed milk, plus extra for serving
Sea salt

1. Put the oats, chopped dates and spices into a medium heavy-based saucepan with three-quarters of the apple chunks and add a pinch of salt. Pour in the milk and 400ml of hot water and stir over a medium heat until the porridge begins to simmer.

2. Simmer gently for 15–20 minutes, stirring regularly for a creamy consistency. The apple chunks will collapse into the porridge and the liquid should all be absorbed.

3. To serve, spoon into warmed bowls and top with the remaining apple chunks. Serve with a little jug of extra milk on the side.

PER SERVING	
KCAL	231
FAT (g)	5.0
SATURATES (g)	2.0
CARBS (g)	36.0
SUGARS (g)	15.0
FIBRE (g)	4.0
PROTEIN (g)	8.0
SALT (g)	0.23

VARIATIONS
Swap the cow's milk for soya, rice or oat milk, or, for a very lean version, just make it with water.

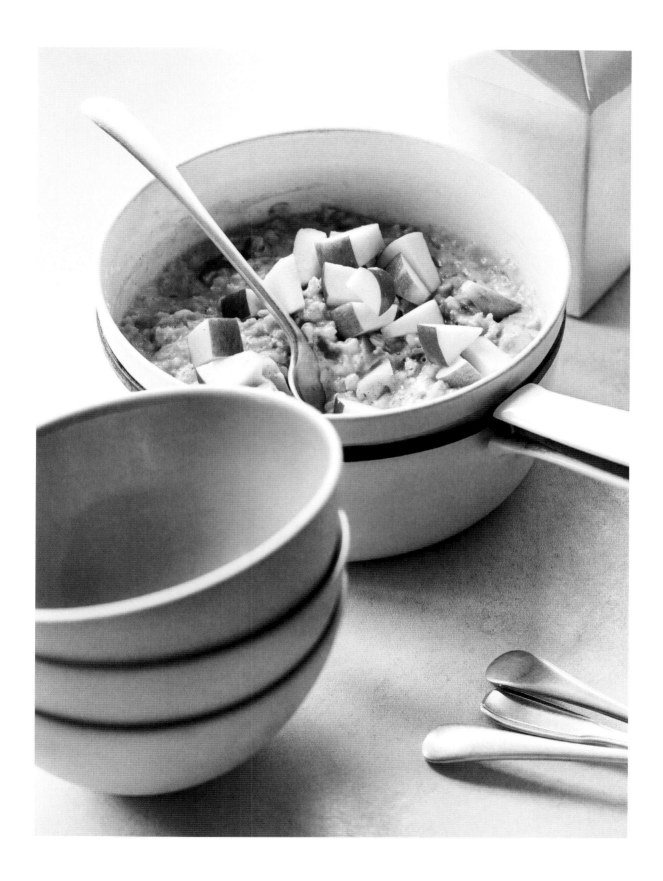

RAINBOW VEGETABLE FRITTATA

SERVES 4

Making a cooked breakfast for the family can be a bit hectic in the morning, with everyone wanting different things, but making a frittata is much less labour-intensive while still satisfying the desire for something hot. It's better for you too – this version is full of healthy veg to get the day off to a good start and, thanks to the protein-rich eggs, would make an ideal post-run brunch. Serve it straight from the grill or at room temperature.

Olive oil, for frying
2 garlic cloves, peeled and finely chopped
1 red pepper, deseeded and sliced
1 orange pepper, deseeded and sliced
1 courgette, cut into small chunks
5 stalks rainbow chard, finely sliced
8 eggs, beaten
Sea salt and freshly ground black pepper

1. Preheat the grill to medium.

2. Heat a dash of oil in a 25cm non-stick, ovenproof frying pan. Gently fry the garlic over a medium heat until just cooked through but not turning golden.

3. Add the peppers and a pinch of salt and sauté for 5–6 minutes, until softened. Add the courgette and cook for a further 2 minutes to soften slightly, then add the chard along with 1 tablespoon of hot water (if using spinach there is no need to add the hot water) and continue to cook for 4–5 minutes, stirring gently, until the chard has wilted.

4. Season the beaten eggs and pour over the vegetables, gently shaking the pan to make sure they are evenly spread out. Cook over a medium-low heat for 5–7 minutes, until the frittata is almost set. Transfer to the grill for a couple of minutes, until the top is golden and the frittata is cooked through.

5. Remove from the grill and loosen the edges of the frittata from the pan. Slide on to a serving board or plate and cut into wedges to serve.

PER SERVING	
KCAL	203
FAT (g)	11.0
SATURATES (g)	3.0
CARBS (g)	6.0
SUGARS (g)	5.0
FIBRE (g)	3.0
PROTEIN (g)	17.0
SALT (g)	0.76

VARIATION
If you can't get hold of rainbow chard, replace it with a handful of Swiss chard, spinach or another green leafy vegetable, such as spring greens or kale, though these will take longer to soften.

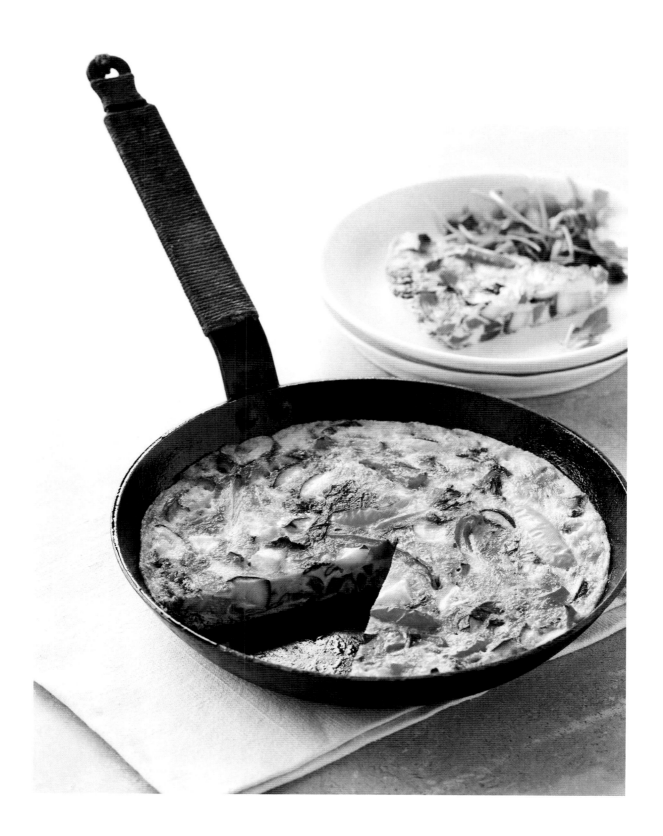

NUTRITIOUS LUNCHES AND SALADS

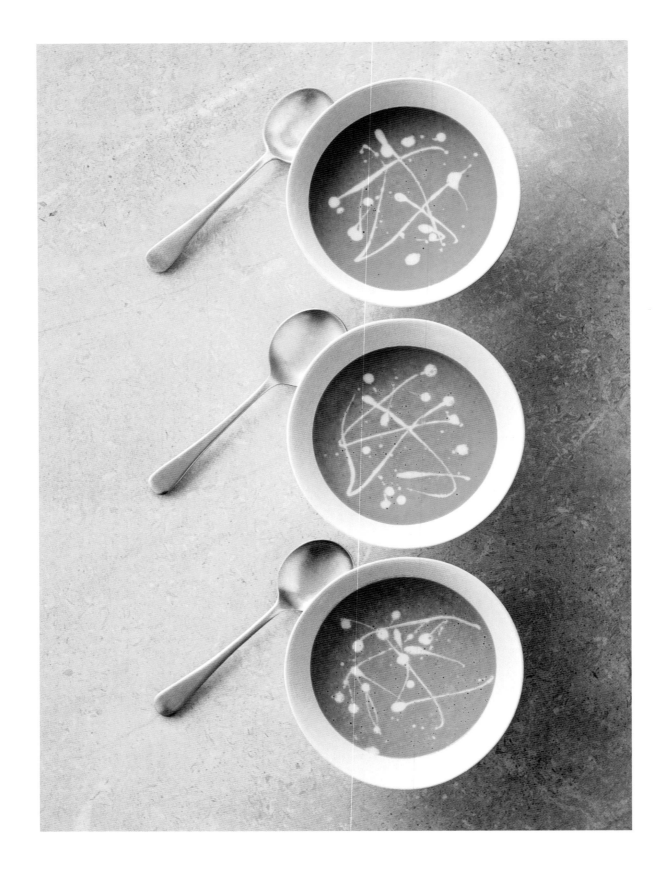

CHILLED PEA AND COCONUT SOUP
SERVES 6

I think that a chilled soup is a very elegant dish to serve at a summer lunch or in shot glasses as a canapé, and this one is really easy to make while still being packed full of flavour and richness, not to mention goodness. If the weather doesn't go your way, it's also good heated up. Coconut milk does contain a lot of saturated fat, so keep an eye on portion sizes here or serve it when you know you are going to be active to use up all the easily metabolized energy it provides (see page 230).

1 x 400ml tin reduced fat coconut milk
400ml coconut water
Juice of 1 lemon
100g spinach leaves, washed
Small bunch of mint, leaves roughly chopped
750g frozen peas, defrosted
2.5cm piece of fresh root ginger, peeled and
  roughly chopped
1 green chilli, deseeded and roughly chopped
Sea salt and freshly ground black pepper

1. Set aside 3 tablespoons of coconut milk, then put all the rest of the ingredients into a blender or food processor with 600ml of water. Add a couple of pinches of salt and pepper and blend until really smooth. Depending on the size of your blender, you may need to do this in batches. If this is the case, divide the ingredients in half and blend together.

2. Taste the soup and adjust the seasoning if necessary.

3. Serve chilled, and stir before serving, drizzled with the reserved coconut milk.

HOW TO SERVE IT WARM
As the flavours in chilled soup can be a little muted, be generous with the seasoning and taste often. On the flip side, if you are serving this soup warm, watch the chilli levels – the effects will be stronger, so add less if you don't like things too hot.

PER SERVING	
KCAL	117
FAT (g)	6.0
SATURATES (g)	5.0
CARBS (g)	17.0
SUGARS (g)	9.0
FIBRE (g)	8.0
PROTEIN (g)	9.0
SALT (g)	0.21

CORONATION CHICKPEAS

SERVES 4

Chickpeas carry spice brilliantly, so they are the base of this vegetarian take on Coronation Chicken. Unlike the classic cold chicken dish, this is not drenched in mayonnaise but is made healthier with a yoghurt-based dressing, and you won't miss the chicken because chickpeas are rich in fibre, which helps fill you up, regulates appetite and reduces cravings. This salad is almost better if you make it in advance, as the flavours really get a chance to meld together, so make it the day before you eat it if you can. Serve with cold basmati rice and a crisp green salad to make a meal of it.

2 x 400g tins chickpeas, drained and rinsed
1 small cauliflower, cut into really small florets
2 carrots, diced
3 spring onions, trimmed and finely chopped

FOR THE DRESSING
200g natural yoghurt
2 tsp curry powder
½ tsp turmeric powder
1 tsp ground cumin
2 tsp cider vinegar
1 tsp Dijon mustard
Sea salt and freshly ground black pepper

1. Put the drained chickpeas, cauliflower florets, carrots and spring onions into a large mixing bowl and toss to mix.

2. In a smaller bowl, mix together the dressing ingredients and season with salt and black pepper.

3. Pour the dressing over the chickpeas and mix really well so that everything is coated. Taste and adjust the seasoning if necessary. Cover and store in the fridge until ready to use. It will last for up to 3 days in the fridge.

PER SERVING	
KCAL	243
FAT (g)	6.0
SATURATES (g)	1.0
CARBS (g)	29.0
SUGARS (g)	9.0
FIBRE (g)	10.0
PROTEIN (g)	14.0
SALT (g)	0.31

ROASTED BUTTERNUT SQUASH, FARRO AND SUMAC SALAD

SERVES 4

Sumac is a citrusy spice that is popular in the Middle East. It lifts the earthy flavours of this salad, counterbalancing the sweetness of the butternut and giving the dish a lemony freshness. It's a great addition to your store cupboard and goes brilliantly wherever you might add a squeeze of lemon. Farro is a grain similar to pearl barley that is nutty and chewy when cooked. Though wheat has got a bad name for itself in these gluten-fearing times, these unprocessed whole grains are an excellent source of fibre, protein and energizing B vitamins and they turn this salad into a substantial meal.

1 large butternut squash, peeled, halved lengthways and deseeded
4 garlic cloves, bashed but not peeled
Olive oil, for drizzling
1 tsp sumac, plus extra for sprinkling
200g farro
100g kale, chopped into bite-sized pieces
30g flaked almonds, toasted
Sea salt and freshly ground black pepper

FOR THE DRESSING
Juice of 1 lemon
2 tbsp tahini
½ tsp sumac
½ tsp runny honey

CONTINUED OVERLEAF

PER SERVING	
KCAL	367
FAT (g)	13.0
SATURATES (g)	2.0
CARBS (g)	43.0
SUGARS (g)	11.0
FIBRE (g)	10.0
PROTEIN (g)	14.0
SALT (g)	0.05

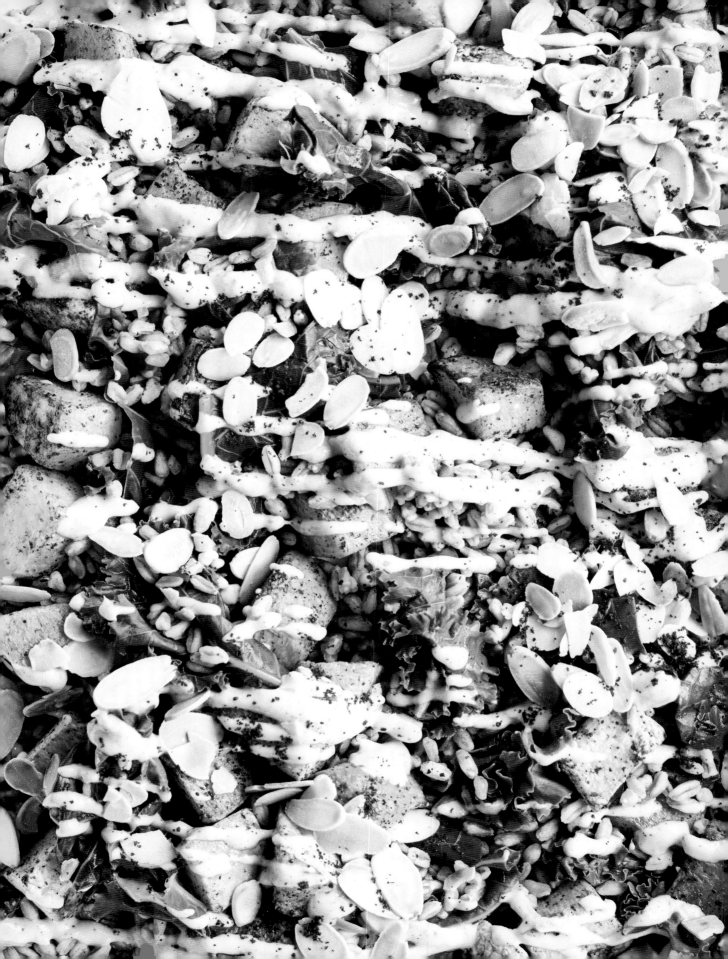

CONTINUED FROM PAGE 45

1. Preheat the oven to 200°C/gas 6.

2. Cut the butternut squash into 2cm cubes. Put them into a roasting tin with the bashed garlic cloves and drizzle with a little olive oil. Season with salt and pepper and sprinkle over the teaspoon of sumac. Toss to coat evenly, then place in the preheated oven and cook for 30–35 minutes, until soft and lightly browned on the edges.

3. Meanwhile, bring a pan of water to the boil and add the farro. Simmer over a medium-low heat for 20–30 minutes, until the farro is tender but with a slight bite. For the last 5 minutes of the cooking time, add the kale to the pan and stir through.

4. Once the kale and farro are cooked, remove from the heat, drain and leave to cool.

5. When the butternut squash is ready, remove the tray from the oven. Pick out the garlic and squeeze the flesh out of the skins into a small mixing bowl. Mash the garlic with the back of a fork and add the dressing ingredients with a pinch of salt and pepper. Mix together really well with a fork to combine, then drizzle in 1 tablespoon of water, stirring continuously.

6. Put the farro, kale and butternut squash into a large serving bowl and toss gently to mix together. Drizzle over the dressing and sprinkle with the toasted flaked almonds and a little extra sumac. Serve immediately or store in the fridge for up to 4 days. Toss well before serving.

VARIATIONS
You can substitute pumpkin, sweet potatoes or carrots for the butternut squash. And if you can't get hold of farro it can be replaced with spelt, freekeh or bulgur wheat. This salad would also be delicious with the addition of spoonfuls of ricotta or goat's cheese dotted on top.

ROASTED CAULIFLOWER, QUINOA AND POMEGRANATE SALAD

SERVES 4

Roasting brassicas like cauliflower, broccoli, kale and cabbage intensifies the flavour and they become sweet and almost caramelized around the edges. Cooking cauliflower this way and tossing it in this sharp pomegranate molasses dressing might just convert a few cauliflower-haters to the cause. It's a vibrant, satisfying salad that works really well with slow-cooked lamb, chargrilled chicken or halloumi.

1 large cauliflower, cut into florets
Olive oil, for drizzling
200g quinoa, rinsed
Small bunch of flat-leaf parsley, leaves picked
Seeds from 1 pomegranate

FOR THE DRESSING
1 tbsp pomegranate molasses
1 tbsp white wine vinegar
1 garlic clove, peeled and crushed
6 tbsp extra virgin olive oil
Sea salt and freshly ground black pepper

1. Preheat the oven to 190°C/gas 5.

2. Place the cauliflower florets on a baking tray and drizzle with a little olive oil. Season with salt and pepper and toss in the oil to coat. Transfer to the preheated oven and roast for 20 minutes, turning the cauliflower halfway through, until browned in places. Remove from the oven once cooked.

3. Meanwhile, cook the quinoa according to the packet instructions. Drain off any excess water.

4. Using a small whisk or a fork, mix the ingredients for the dressing together with a pinch of salt and pepper until completely combined. Taste and adjust the seasoning if necessary.

5. Put the cooked quinoa and the cauliflower into a large mixing bowl. Drizzle with the dressing and fold in the parsley leaves. Scatter over the pomegranate seeds to serve.

PER SERVING	
KCAL	386
FAT (g)	21.0
SATURATES (g)	3.0
CARBS (g)	36.0
SUGARS (g)	10.0
FIBRE (g)	7.0
PROTEIN (g)	11.0
SALT (g)	0.11

GOOD TO KNOW
Pomegranate seeds are bursting with vitamin C, which boosts your immune system, and vitamin K, which is essential for bone and blood health. As well as fighting bacteria, supporting the heart and lowering blood pressure, they are also supposed to be aphrodisiacs!

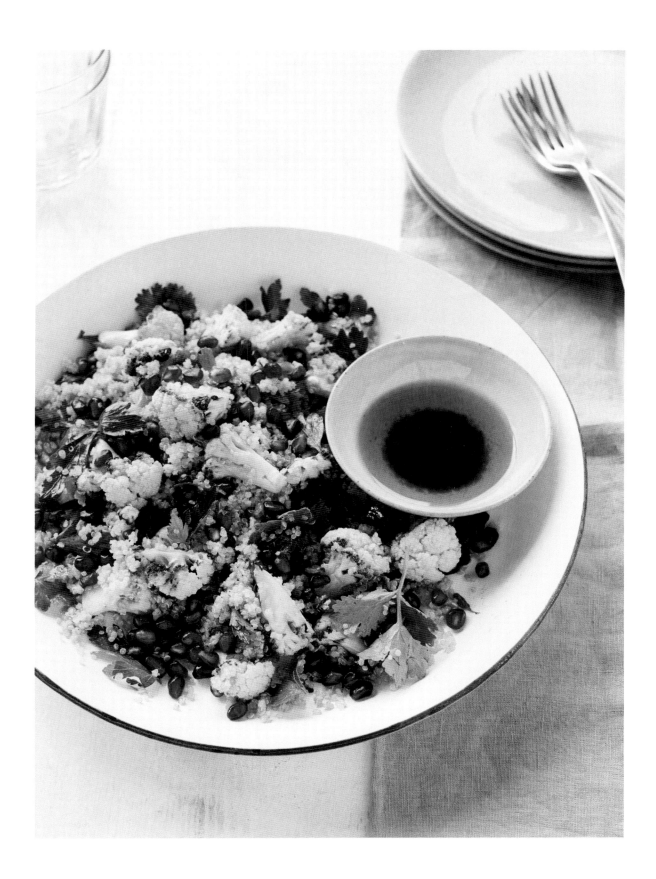

ADUKI BEAN, SWEET POTATO AND FENNEL SALAD

SERVES 4

This is my kind of salad – it's substantial and tasty and has a great combination of earthy colours and flavours. Furthermore, thanks to the protein in the beans and quinoa, it will fill you up for the rest of the afternoon. It's delicious served warm but is just as good cold, so can be made in advance or even the night before.

2 medium sweet potatoes, scrubbed clean
    and cubed
Olive oil, for roasting and frying
200g kale, stalks removed and leaves
    chopped into bite-sized pieces
1 garlic clove, peeled and finely chopped
60g rocket leaves
1 x 400g tin aduki beans, drained
    and rinsed
250g cooked quinoa (from approximately
    85g uncooked quinoa)
1 large fennel bulb, diced
Sea salt and freshly ground black pepper

FOR THE DRESSING
1 garlic clove, peeled and crushed
1½ tbsp cider vinegar
1 heaped tsp Dijon mustard
Juice of ½ orange
½ tsp dried chilli flakes (optional)
4½ tbsp extra virgin olive oil

1. Preheat the oven to 180°C/gas 4.

2. Toss the cubed sweet potatoes in a little oil and season with salt and pepper. Spread in a single layer on a baking tray and place in the preheated oven for 30 minutes, turning halfway through.

3. Meanwhile, place a frying pan over a medium heat and add a dash of oil. When hot, add the kale with a pinch of salt and 2 tablespoons of water. Sauté for 2 minutes, until the kale has wilted and the water has evaporated. Add the garlic and stir through. Continue to cook for a further 2 minutes, until the garlic has softened.

4. In a large salad bowl, whisk together the garlic, vinegar, mustard, orange juice and chilli flakes, if using. Season with a pinch of salt and pepper, then slowly pour in the extra virgin olive oil, whisking continuously until emulsified. Taste and adjust the flavours as necessary.

5. Put the rocket into the bowl, then add the aduki beans, quinoa, roasted sweet potato and kale and gently mix together. Scatter over the diced fennel before serving.

PER SERVING	
KCAL	447
FAT (g)	16.0
SATURATES (g)	2.0
CARBS (g)	55.0
SUGARS (g)	15.0
FIBRE (g)	13.0
PROTEIN (g)	13.0
SALT (g)	0.36

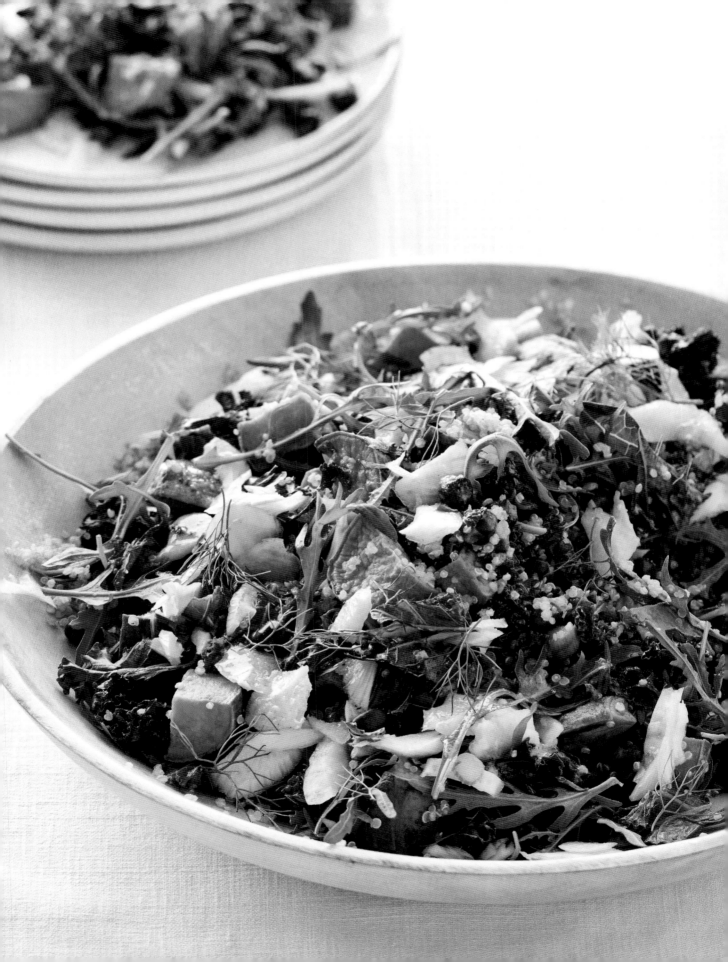

SOUTH-EAST-ASIAN-INSPIRED NOODLE SALAD

SERVES 4

Tana loves noodle salads full of crunchy veg, nuts and fresh herbs, with that unmistakable Asian-style dressing made of lime, fish sauce and chilli, so there is often a big bowl made up in the fridge at home. I'm also a fan, as they are light yet filling and full of crunch and flavour. You could stir through some shredded poached chicken or batons of mozzarella to add extra protein.

200g brown rice vermicelli noodles
100g roasted, unsalted peanuts, roughly chopped
3 carrots
1 medium cucumber, julienned
100g radishes, trimmed and sliced
2 spring onions, trimmed and finely chopped
Large bunch of coriander, stalks and
  leaves chopped
Small bunch of mint, leaves roughly torn

FOR THE DRESSING
Juice of 4 limes
2 tsp agave syrup
1 tbsp fish sauce, to taste
½ long red chilli, deseeded and finely chopped
  (optional)

PER SERVING	
KCAL	386
FAT (g)	13.0
SATURATES (g)	2.0
CARBS (g)	51.0
SUGARS (g)	10.0
FIBRE (g)	6.0
PROTEIN (g)	14.0
SALT (g)	0.83

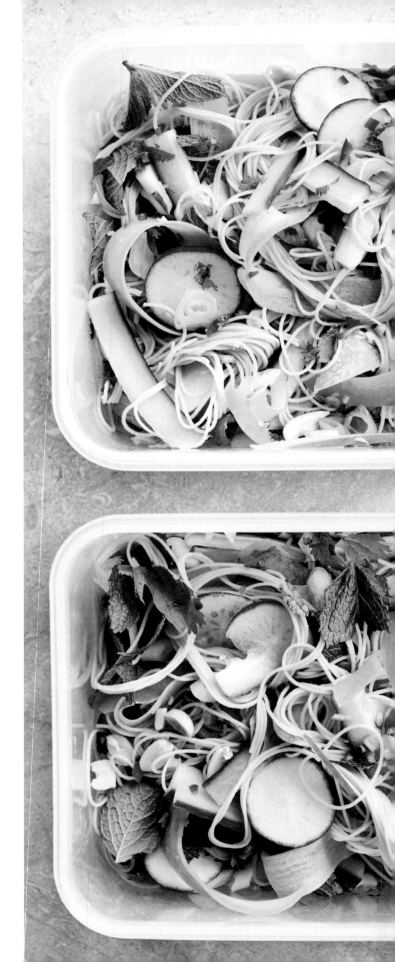

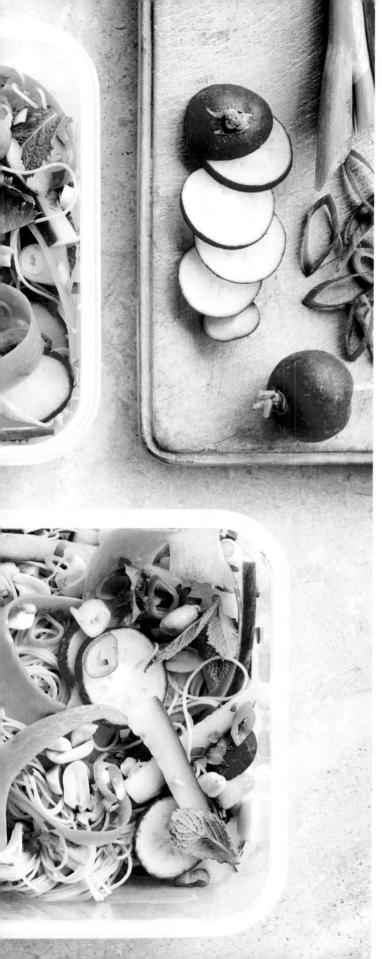

1. Soak the noodles according to their packet instructions. Once soft, drain and run under cold water to cool.

2. Toast the peanuts in a dry frying pan over a medium heat until lightly golden.

3. Using a vegetable peeler, peel the carrots into ribbons and put them into the bowl with the cooled noodles. Add the cucumber, radishes, spring onions, coriander and mint to the bowl and toss really well to mix everything together.

4. For the dressing, mix together the lime juice, agave syrup, fish sauce and chilli, if using, then taste to check the balance (see below). Adjust the flavours as necessary.

5. Pour the dressing over the salad and add the toasted peanuts. Mix well, then serve or store covered in the fridge for up to 3 days.

HOW TO BALANCE THE DRESSING

For the dressing, you are aiming for a balance between sweet, salty, spicy and sour, with no one ingredient being more pronounced than the other. For example, if you can taste lime juice more than any other ingredient, add a little more agave and/or fish sauce, and likewise with the other ingredients.

PRAWN WALDORF SALAD

SERVES 4

A classic Waldorf salad is a combination of crunchy apple, grapes, celery and walnuts, which would be really good for you if it wasn't then coated with a thick layer of mayonnaise. Here I've added prawns for extra protein and swapped the calorie-rich mayo for a much lighter Greek yoghurt dressing, so you can have your Waldorf salad and eat it, after all. The celery heart is the more tender inner stalks of the head that are often sold separately.

75g walnuts
1 small romaine lettuce, finely shredded
200g cooked, peeled king prawns, deveined
   if necessary
1 celery heart, chopped
1 eating apple e.g. Granny Smith, cored and
   cut into 1cm pieces
100g seedless green grapes, washed and halved

FOR THE DRESSING
100g Greek yoghurt
1½ tsp Dijon mustard
1 tsp cider vinegar
Juice of ½ lemon
Sea salt and freshly ground black pepper

1. Start by making the dressing; whisk together all the ingredients in a small mixing bowl. Taste and adjust the seasoning as necessary, adding a little more lemon juice if required.

2. Toast the walnuts in a dry frying pan over a medium heat for 2–3 minutes until golden.

3. Put the shredded lettuce leaves into a large mixing bowl and add the prawns, celery, apple and grapes. Spoon in the dressing and toss to coat. Taste and adjust the seasoning as necessary before serving.

PER SERVING	
KCAL	258
FAT (g)	16.0
SATURATES (g)	3.0
CARBS (g)	10.0
SUGARS (g)	10.0
FIBRE (g)	4.0
PROTEIN (g)	15.0
SALT (g)	1.14

SALAD TO GO
If you are taking this salad to work or on a picnic, dress it in the morning but don't add the lettuce until you are ready to eat it.

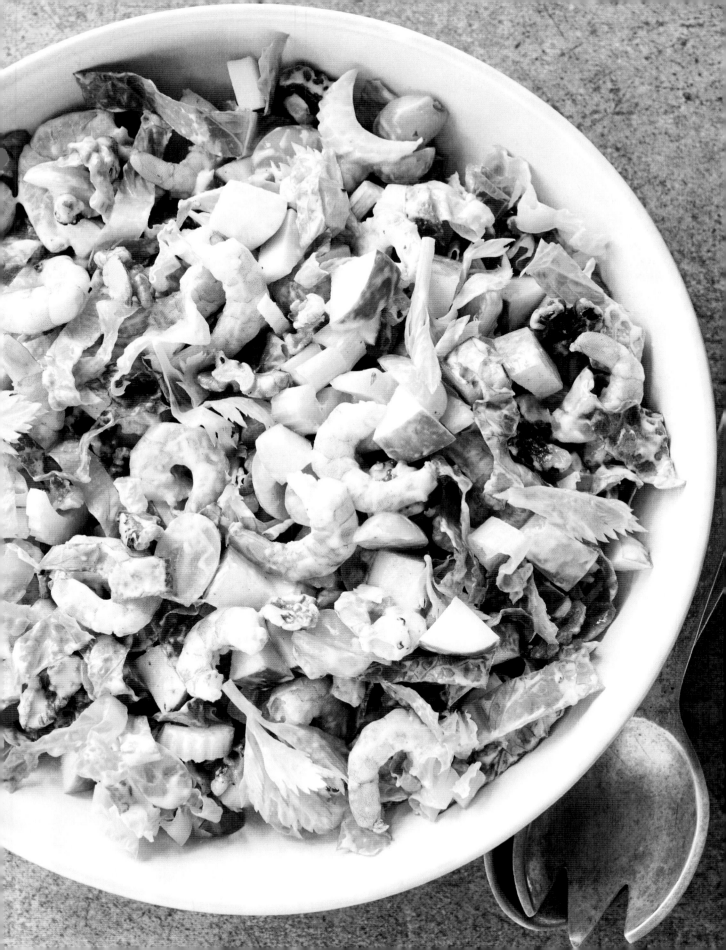

TUNA AND AVOCADO TARTARE

SERVES 4

Tuna tartare looks really sophisticated and impressive, but you can pull it all together in a matter of minutes. Tuna is one of the oily fish, full of omega-3 fatty acids, that we are advised to eat at least once a week, and this makes a perfect light lunch with a green salad on the side. Make sure you get sushi grade tuna which is as fresh as possible, and don't assemble the dish until just before you are ready to eat it, otherwise the lime juice will 'cook' the fish and turn it brown. Serve with a rocket salad and Pitta Crisps (see page 266) to scoop up the tuna.

2 tsp white or black sesame seeds
Small bunch of chives, very finely chopped
1 tbsp soy sauce
Juice of 1 lime
½ tsp sesame oil
400g tuna steak, finely chopped
1 large ripe avocado, peeled, stoned and diced
Sea salt and freshly ground black pepper

1. Place a small frying pan over a low heat and toast the white sesame seeds until golden and aromatic, then leave to cool. (There is no need to toast black sesame seeds.)

2. Put the chives, soy sauce, half the lime juice and the sesame oil into a mixing bowl. Add the tuna, season with a little salt and pepper and toss to coat.

3. Put the avocado into another mixing bowl and gently fold in the remaining lime juice.

4. Divide the tuna between four plates, making a small mound of it in the centre. Spoon the avocado on top, then sprinkle with sesame seeds and serve immediately (see below).

PER SERVING	
KCAL	224
FAT (g)	12.0
SATURATES (g)	3.0
CARBS (g)	2.0
SUGARS (g)	1.0
FIBRE (g)	3.0
PROTEIN (g)	27.0
SALT (g)	0.69

HOW TO DRESS THIS UP
To plate this as we do in the restaurant, rub the inside of a 6–8cm round pastry ring with a little extra sesame oil and place it in the centre of a serving plate. Spoon in a quarter of the tuna tartare, add a quarter of the diced avocado on top and sprinkle with sesame seeds, then gently and slowly remove the ring.

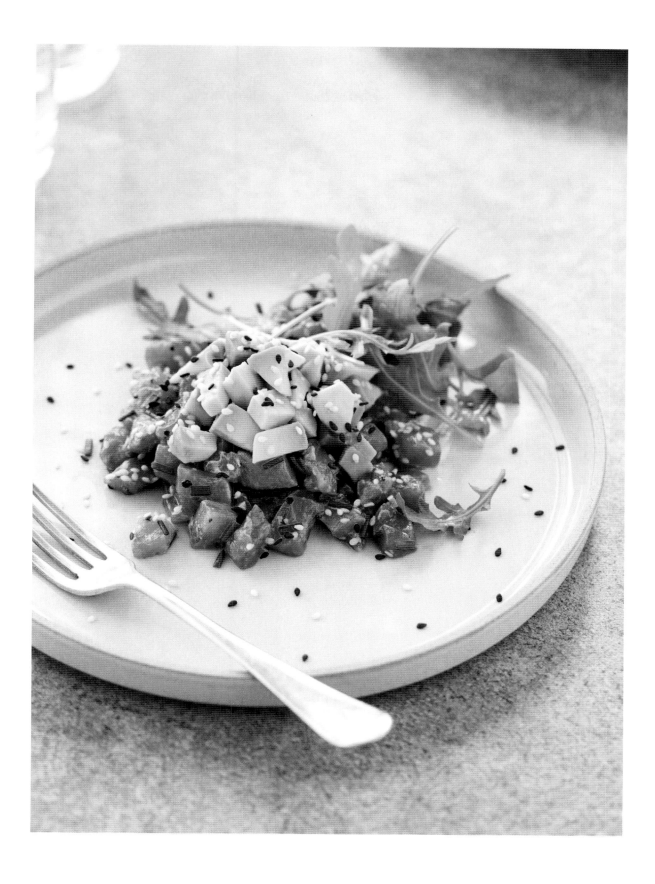

HEALTHY VEGETABLE SAMOSAS

SERVES 4 (MAKES 16 SAMOSAS)

'Healthy' and 'samosa' aren't two words I'd expect to see in the same sentence, but these are samosas with a difference . . . They are made with rice paper spring roll wrappers rather than the traditional fatty pastry, then baked in the oven rather than fried so they don't absorb all that oil during the cooking. They're stuffed full of vegetables too, so as samosas go these really are as healthy as they can be. My kids love them, so we make up big batches for after-school snacks for them and their friends.

1½ tsp garam masala
1½ tsp ground cumin
1½ tsp ground coriander
1½ tsp black mustard seeds
1 tbsp coconut oil, plus extra for brushing
1 onion, peeled and diced
1 garlic clove, peeled and finely chopped
2.5cm piece of fresh root ginger, peeled and grated
1 small cauliflower, cut into very small florets about 1cm
1 carrot, finely chopped into 1cm cubes
100g frozen peas, defrosted
16 rice paper wrappers
Sea salt and freshly ground black pepper

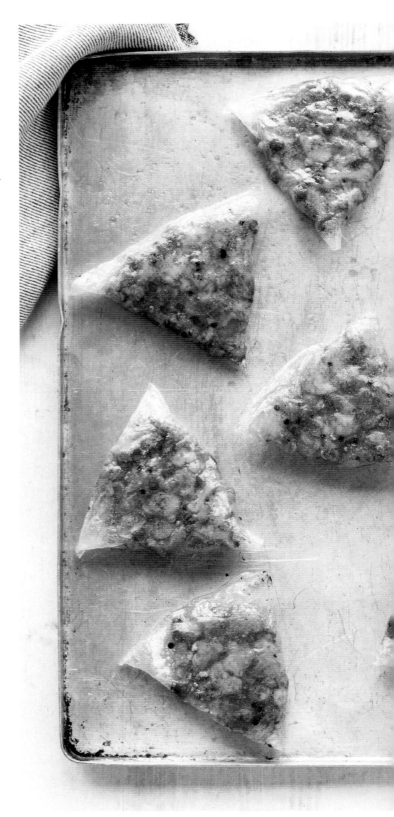

PER SERVING	
KCAL	254
FAT (g)	5.0
SATURATES (g)	3.0
CARBS (g)	42.0
SUGARS (g)	8.0
FIBRE (g)	5.0
PROTEIN (g)	7.0
SALT (g)	1.14

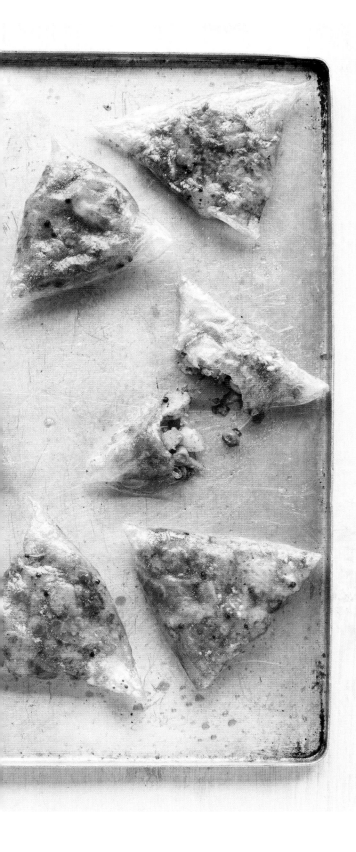

1. Preheat the oven to 200°C/gas 6.

2. Place a large frying pan over a medium heat and add the spices. Toast for 30 seconds or until aromatic, then add the coconut oil, diced onion and a pinch of salt. Turn the heat down a little and sauté for 6–8 minutes, until soft.

3. Stir in the garlic and ginger and cook for a further 2 minutes. Add the cauliflower and carrots and 100ml of hot water. Turn the heat up a little and bring the water to the boil, stirring the vegetables until tender but still with a slight crunch (about 4–5 minutes).

4. Once the water has evaporated, add the peas and cook for a further 2–3 minutes. Taste and adjust the seasoning as necessary, then remove from the heat and leave to cool.

5. Once ready to assemble the samosas, fill a shallow dish with warm water. Dip a rice paper wrapper into the water and leave until it becomes just pliable (don't let it get too waterlogged, as this will cause it to rip). Place the softened rice paper wrapper on a board and fold it in half to create a half-moon shape with the curved side to the right.

6. Place a heaped tablespoon of the mixture in the middle of the half-moon. Fold the bottom corner over the mixture two-thirds of the way up the curved side. Fold down the top corner to enclose the mixture, then fold over the edges to seal. The rice paper should still be wet enough to stick, but if it isn't, put a little water on your finger and run it along the edges before you fold and seal them. Repeat with the remaining mixture and rice paper wrappers.

7. Place the samosas on a baking tray with the sealed edges facing downwards and brush each of them with a little coconut oil. Put the tray into the preheated oven and bake for 10 minutes.

8. Remove from the oven, gently turn each of the samosas over and brush the side facing up with a little more coconut oil. Return to the oven and cook for a further 10 minutes.

9. Remove from the oven and eat while hot, or leave to cool and take on a picnic or packed lunch.

SUPER SUPPERS AND SIDES

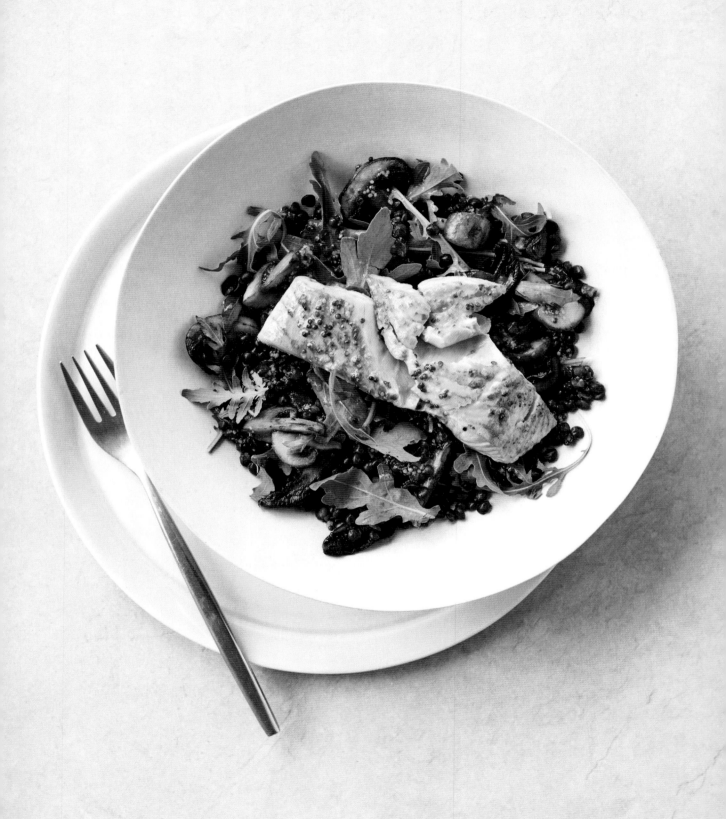

GRILLED SALMON WITH GARLIC MUSHROOM AND LENTIL SALAD

SERVES 4

Winter salad may sound like a contradiction in terms, but this combination of lentils, mushrooms and rocket is just that. It's a hearty, robust dish, perfect for autumnal and wintry days when regular salad ingredients are out of season. It's delicious on its own but is particularly good with grilled wild salmon, which also adds extra protein, healthy fats and plenty of vitamins and minerals to your meal.

200g Puy lentils
1 bay leaf
2 thyme sprigs
800ml vegetable stock (or water)
1 tbsp olive oil
200g chestnut mushrooms, cut into eighths
200g large flat or Portobello mushrooms, sliced
2 garlic cloves, peeled and finely chopped
4 x 100g wild salmon fillets
100g rocket leaves
Sea salt and freshly ground black pepper

FOR THE DRESSING
1 garlic clove, peeled and crushed
2 tbsp white wine vinegar
1 tsp wholegrain mustard
1 tsp runny honey
1 tbsp extra virgin olive oil
1 tbsp water

1. Put the lentils into a large saucepan along with the bay leaf, thyme and stock (or water). Bring to the boil over a medium–high heat, then reduce to a simmer. Simmer for 15–20 minutes until tender.

2. In the meantime, heat a large heavy-based frying pan over a medium–high heat and add the olive oil. Once hot, add the mushrooms with a pinch of salt and cook in the pan for 6–8 minutes, stirring now and again, until soft and lightly caramelized on the edges.

3. Add the chopped garlic and continue to cook for 2 minutes, then remove the pan from the heat.

4. Once the lentils are tender, drain well and discard the herbs. Put the lentils into a large mixing bowl and add the mushrooms. Mix together gently to avoid breaking up the lentils too much.

5. To make the dressing, put all the ingredients into a clean jam jar with a pinch of salt and pepper. Close the lid of the jar and shake until the dressing comes together and emulsifies.

6. Preheat the grill to high. Grill the salmon for 6–8 minutes to your liking.

7. Pour half the dressing over the warm lentils and toss gently to ensure everything is coated. Fold in the rocket, place the salmon on top and pour over the remaining dressing. Serve immediately.

HOW TO SAVE TIME
To shorten the prep time, use pre-cooked lentils in tins or pouches. For four people, you will need 2 x 400g tins or 2–3 pouches.

PER SERVING	
KCAL	480
FAT (g)	20.0
SATURATES (g)	3.0
CARBS (g)	29.0
SUGARS (g)	5.0
FIBRE (g)	9.0
PROTEIN (g)	43.0
SALT (g)	0.78

MISO COD EN PAPILLOTE

SERVES 4

Miso black cod, a Japanese favourite made popular around the world by the restaurant Nobu, is actually made with sable fish, which isn't cod at all. As it's difficult to get hold of in the UK, I've come up with a way of using the same deep flavours with regular cod. This dish is fantastic for entertaining, as you can marinate the fish and make up the parcels in advance, then put them into the oven at the last minute. Let everyone open the parcels at the table so they get to smell the heady miso steam that comes out when they are opened. Serve with steamed rice and stir-fried vegetables.

4 tbsp mirin
2 tbsp white miso paste
1 tbsp maple syrup
2 tsp soy sauce
4 cod fillets (approximately 125g each), skinned and pin-boned
Olive oil, for drizzling
4 pak choi, leaves separated from the stem
4cm piece of fresh root ginger, peeled and cut into matchsticks
4 spring onions, trimmed and finely sliced

1. Mix together the mirin, miso paste, maple syrup and soy sauce in a shallow dish. Add the fish fillets and turn to coat them in the marinade. Cover and leave to marinate in the fridge for at least 4 hours, or up to 2 days.

2. Preheat the oven to 170°C/gas 3.

3. Drizzle four large pieces of foil or baking paper with a little olive oil and place a pile of pak choi leaves in the middle of each square. Top with a layer of ginger and spring onions, then place the cod fillets on top, spooning over any remaining marinade.

4. Draw the edges of the foil or paper together, fold over to make a parcel and seal tightly, leaving room for steam to circulate. Place the parcels on a baking tray.

5. Bake in the preheated oven for 10–12 minutes until the fish is just cooked through.

6. Remove and leave to rest for a few minutes before putting each parcel on to a plate for your guests to open themselves.

PER SERVING	
KCAL	171
FAT (g)	1.0
SATURATES (g)	0.1
CARBS (g)	15.0
SUGARS (g)	10.0
FIBRE (g)	3.0
PROTEIN (g)	24.0
SALT (g)	1.35

GOOD TO KNOW
As well as being delicious and nutritious, this dish is also low in fat so an excellent recipe for when you are watching your weight.

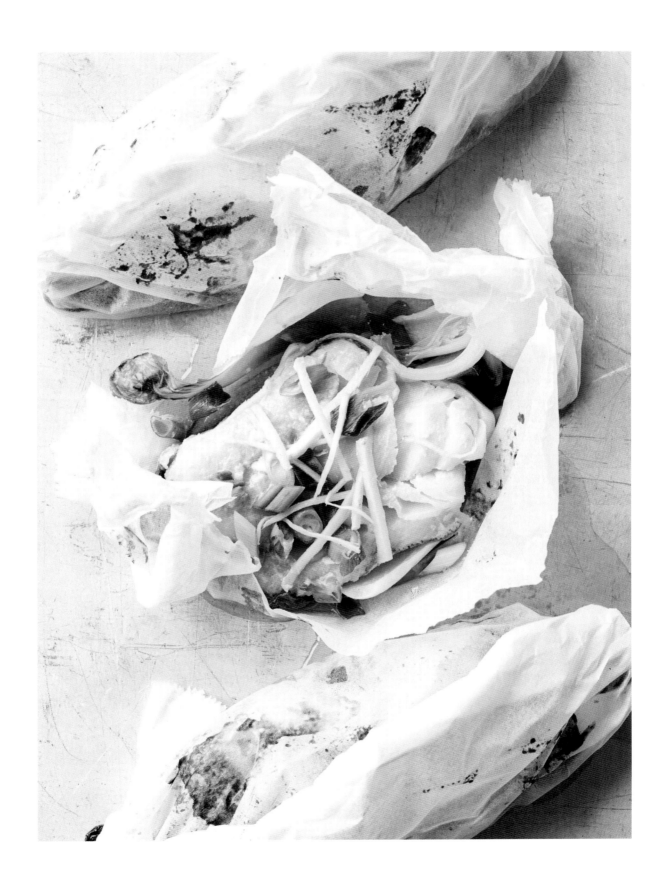

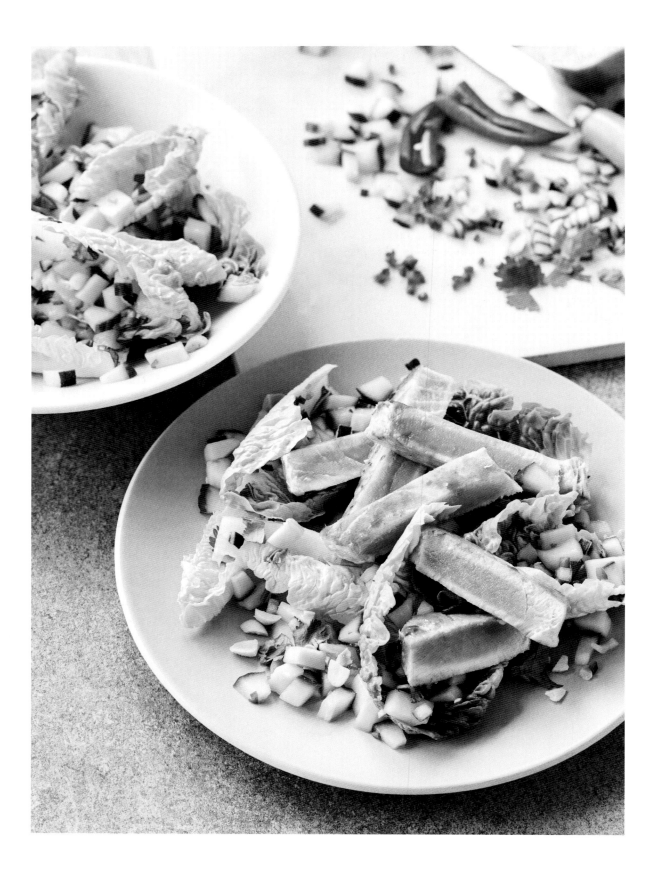

TUNA STEAK WITH MANGO AND CUCUMBER SALSA

SERVES 2

Oily fish like fresh tuna are full of vital omega-3 fatty acids that are said to protect the heart as well as lowering blood pressure and reducing fat build-up in the arteries. These essential fats are considered so good for you that the UK government recommends we eat at least one portion of oily fish every week. If you have fish-avoiding children, meaty tuna is a really good way to bring them round, especially when served with this delicious salsa – just leave out the chilli if they don't like spice.

1 small mango, peeled and finely diced
1 small red onion, peeled and finely diced
½ cucumber, diced
Small bunch of coriander, roughly chopped
Small bunch of basil, roughly chopped
25g unsalted peanuts, roughly chopped
1 red chilli, deseeded and finely chopped
2 tsp fish sauce
Juice of 2 limes
Olive oil, for drizzling
2 tuna steaks (approximately 175g each)
2 baby gem lettuce, leaves separated and washed
Sea salt and freshly ground black pepper

1. Mix the diced mango with the onion, cucumber, coriander, basil, peanuts and red chilli. Pour in the fish sauce and lime juice and mix everything together. Taste and adjust the seasoning as necessary.

2. Drizzle a little olive oil over the tuna steaks and rub it into both sides of the fish. Season with salt and pepper.

3. Place a heavy-based non-stick frying pan over a high heat. When hot, carefully put the fish into the pan and cook for 50 seconds on each side. Remove the fish from the pan and leave to rest for a couple of minutes.

4. Gently toss the baby gem leaves through the salsa and pile up on to two plates. Slice the tuna steaks thickly, then place on top of the leaves and serve.

PER SERVING	
KCAL	416
FAT (g)	13.0
SATURATES (g)	2.0
CARBS (g)	18.0
SUGARS (g)	15.0
FIBRE (g)	6.0
PROTEIN (g)	54.0
SALT (g)	1.36

FILLET STEAK WITH BUTTER BEAN AND FENNEL PURÉE

SERVES 2

Being healthy doesn't mean compromising on flavour. Take this knockout way of serving steak with a rich, velvety purée, intense oyster mushrooms and crispy kale – it's as impressive as it is delicious. Serve it up for a special birthday or anniversary, or increase the quantities for a dinner party and no one will even realize how healthy their food is as they tuck in.

½ tbsp rapeseed oil, plus extra for frying
2 large banana shallots, peeled and diced
2 fennel bulbs, trimmed and roughly chopped into 1cm pieces
1 fresh bay leaf
150ml semi-skimmed milk
250ml chicken stock
1 x 400g tin butter beans, drained and rinsed

75g kale leaves
Olive oil, for drizzling
2 fillet steaks (approximately 150g each)
150g oyster mushrooms, roughly torn into 1cm strips
½ small bunch of parsley, roughly chopped
Juice of ½ lemon
Sea salt and freshly ground black pepper

CONTINUED OVERLEAF

PER SERVING	
KCAL	488
FAT (g)	18.0
SATURATES (g)	5.0
CARBS (g)	24.0
SUGARS (g)	10.0
FIBRE (g)	16.0
PROTEIN (g)	50.0
SALT (g)	0.69

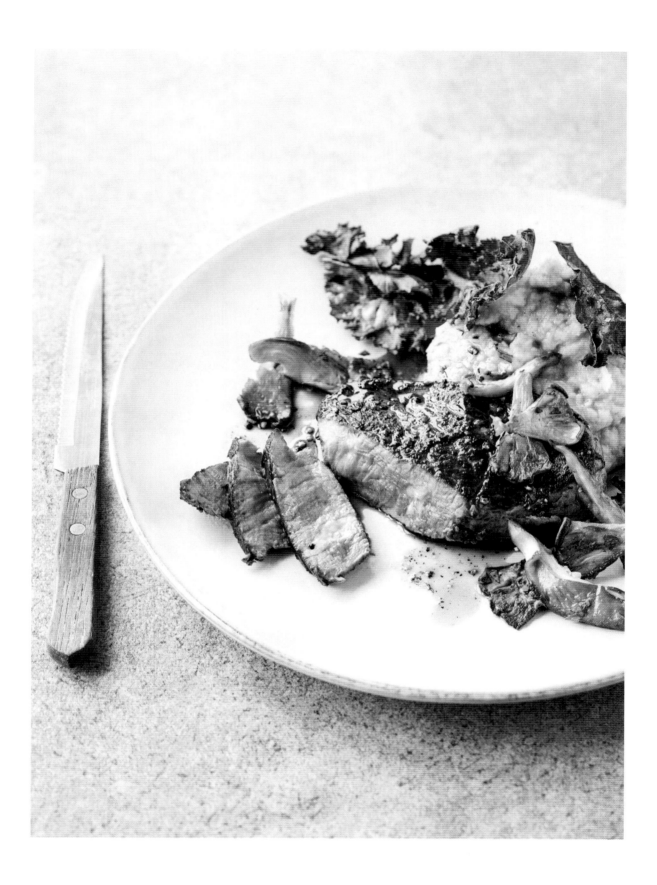

CONTINUED FROM PAGE 68

1. Preheat your oven to 160°C/gas 3.

2. Place a saucepan over a medium-high heat and add the rapeseed oil. When hot, add the shallots, fennel and bay leaf and sweat for 8 minutes.

3. Pour in the milk and chicken stock and bring to the boil, then reduce to a simmer and cook for 10 minutes, until the fennel is soft.

4. Add the butter beans and continue to cook for 10 minutes, until everything is very soft.

5. Meanwhile, toss the kale leaves with a drizzle of olive oil and season with a small pinch of salt. Lay the leaves in a single layer on a baking tray and place in the oven for 15 minutes, or until crisp. Remove and leave to cool.

6. Remove the bay leaf from the fennel and beans and pour the contents of the pan into a blender. Season with salt and blitz until smooth. If the purée isn't loose enough, add a little water and blend again.

7. Brush the steaks with a little rapeseed oil and season all over with salt and pepper. Place a large frying pan over a high heat and, when smoking, carefully add the steaks to the pan and sear all over.

8. Transfer the steaks to a baking tray and roast in the oven for 8 minutes for medium-rare. Remove the steaks from the oven, cover with tin foil and leave to rest in a warm place for 10 minutes.

9. While the steaks are resting, add a little more oil to the same frying pan and place it over a medium-high heat. When hot, add the mushrooms and fry, stirring occasionally, for 3 minutes, until tender and lightly golden. Turn the heat off, season the mushrooms with a little salt and pepper, toss through the chopped parsley and finish with a squeeze of lemon juice.

10. Serve the purée on two warmed plates and place the steaks on the side. Garnish with mushrooms and a handful of kale crisps.

BUTTERNUT SQUASH SPAGHETTI WITH SAGE AND WALNUT PESTO

SERVES 4

Making 'spaghetti' out of pumpkin, sweet potatoes, courgettes or squash is such a good way to increase your veg intake and it looks brilliant too. The sage and walnut pesto can be used with lots of other dishes so make a double batch and keep it in the fridge for up to a week. It's great with chicken, guinea fowl or pork as well as roasted vegetables or stirred into a risotto.

1 large butternut squash
Olive oil, for frying
1 garlic clove, peeled and finely chopped
Grated Parmesan cheese, to serve (optional)

FOR THE SAGE AND WALNUT PESTO
6 sage sprigs, leaves only
½ small bunch of flat-leaf parsley, leaves only
1 garlic clove, peeled and roughly chopped
75g walnuts
Juice of ½ lemon
6 tbsp extra virgin olive oil
Sea salt and freshly ground black pepper

1. Start by making the pesto; put the sage, parsley, garlic and walnuts into a small food processor and blitz until finely chopped.

2. Add the lemon juice and olive oil, season with salt and pepper and blend until emulsified (add a little warm water if the consistency is too thick). Taste and adjust the seasoning as necessary.

3. To make the butternut squash spaghetti, cut off the bulb at the bottom of the squash (save this for soup or the Roasted Butternut Squash, Farro and Sumac Salad on page 45) and the stalk at the top. Peel the remaining part of the squash and use a spiralizer, julienne peeler or mandolin to turn the butternut squash into spaghetti (see below).

4. Place a large frying pan over a medium heat and add a dash of olive oil. Add the chopped garlic and cook for 1 minute then add the squash spaghetti. Toss over the medium heat for 4–5 minutes, until tender but with a slight bite, then remove from the heat and season with salt and pepper.

5. Stir in the pesto and transfer to warm serving bowls to serve. Sprinkle with grated Parmesan, if using.

HOW TO MAKE VEGETABLE SPAGHETTI
You can make vegetable spaghetti really easily with a piece of kit called a spiralizer. These are not expensive and are readily available online, but if you don't want to invest, use a julienne peeler or a mandolin with a julienne attachment. Just be careful of your fingers! For this recipe, try to buy a squash that has a long neck and smaller bottom (where the seeds are), as the neck part is what is used to make the spaghetti.

PER SERVING	
KCAL	359
FAT (g)	31.0
SATURATES (g)	4.0
CARBS (g)	13.0
SUGARS (g)	7.0
FIBRE (g)	4.0
PROTEIN (g)	5.0
SALT (g)	0.02

COURGETTE SPAGHETTI WITH MEATBALLS

SERVES 4

What we call courgetti in the UK, the Americans call zoodles (zucchini noodles) – both great names for this delicious veg 'pasta', which is growing in popularity on both sides of the Atlantic. Courgetti with meatballs is filling and comforting, like a normal bowl of spaghetti, but it's particularly brilliant for all the family as you are upping your veg intake without compromising on flavour or texture. Courgetti is also great with pesto and other classic pasta sauces.

4 large courgettes, trimmed
Olive oil, for frying
Grated Parmesan cheese, to serve (optional)

FOR THE MEATBALLS
500g lean turkey mince
1 small onion, peeled and very finely chopped
2 garlic cloves, peeled and very finely chopped
2 tsp Worcestershire sauce
1 egg, beaten
Sea salt and freshly ground black pepper

FOR THE TOMATO SAUCE
Olive oil, for frying
1 onion, peeled and diced
2 garlic cloves, peeled and crushed
1 tbsp tomato purée
2 x 400g tins chopped tomatoes
½ tsp dried oregano
½ tsp balsamic vinegar

PER SERVING	
KCAL	291
FAT (g)	7.0
SATURATES (g)	1.0
CARBS (g)	16.0
SUGARS (g)	14.0
FIBRE (g)	5.0
PROTEIN (g)	39.0
SALT (g)	0.49

FOR ACTIVE DAYS
Serve the meatballs with wholewheat pasta instead of courgetti if you are gearing up for a big day of exercise.

1. Using a spiralizer (see tip on page 71), julienne peeler or mandolin, turn the 4 courgettes into spaghetti. Put to one side until ready to cook.

2. Put the turkey mince into a mixing bowl with the chopped onion, garlic, Worcestershire sauce, beaten egg and a good pinch of salt and pepper. Mix everything together until thoroughly combined.

3. With wet hands, roll the mixture into 20 meatballs and put them on to a plate. Cover with cling film and chill in the fridge for 30 minutes.

4. Meanwhile, make the tomato sauce. Place a large frying pan over a medium heat and add a dash of olive oil. Once hot, add the onion and sauté for 5–6 minutes until soft, then add the garlic and cook for a further minute.

5. Stir in the tomato purée and continue to cook for 2 minutes, then add the chopped tomatoes, oregano, balsamic vinegar and a good pinch of salt and pepper. Stir everything together and leave to simmer for 10 minutes, until slightly thickened.

6. To cook the meatballs, place a frying pan over a medium heat and add a dash of oil. Once hot, brown the meatballs in batches, turning frequently so they colour on all sides. Transfer to the pan with the tomato sauce to cook for a further 10 minutes until cooked through, turning from time to time. (If the sauce becomes too thick, add 50–100ml of water.)

7. Add an extra teaspoon of oil to the frying pan the meatballs were browned in and gently sauté the courgette spaghetti over a medium heat, tossing occasionally, for 3–5 minutes, until soft but with a slight bite.

8. Divide the courgette spaghetti between serving bowls and top with the meatballs. Sprinkle with Parmesan, if using.

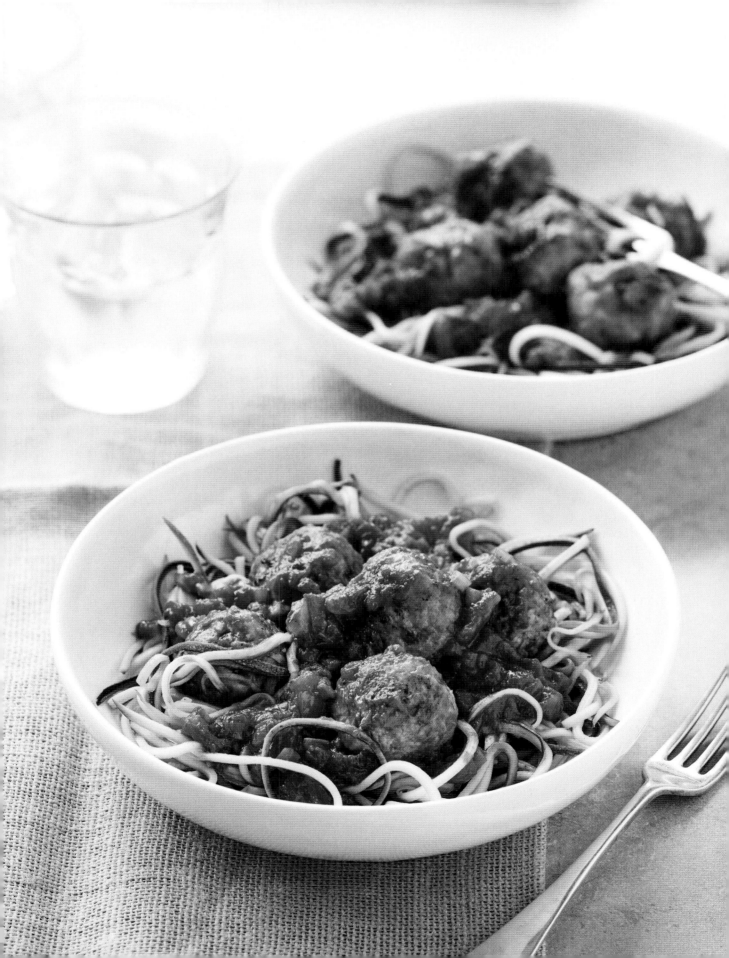

LAMB STEAKS WITH CAULIFLOWER TABBOULEH

SERVES 4

Cauliflower is one of those vegetables that has a bit of a bad reputation. It reminds most people of school dinners and they avoid it unless it's smothered in cheese sauce and grilled. But evidence shows that we should all eat more cauliflower, due to its high levels of vitamin C and folic acid. By blitzing raw cauliflower in a food processor like this, it becomes like rice or couscous, with a crunchy texture that's perfect for a grain-free tabbouleh. (Of course, you can always add some cooked wholewheat couscous or bulgur wheat to this salad if you are in training or building up to a race or match.) This is absolutely delicious with pan-fried lean lamb, halloumi or chicken.

1 medium cauliflower, leaves removed
3 tbsp extra virgin olive oil
250g cherry tomatoes, quartered
1 small red onion, peeled and very finely diced
1 cucumber, finely diced
Large bunch of parsley
Small bunch of mint, leaves picked
Juice of 1 lemon
Rapeseed oil, for frying
4 x 110g lamb leg steaks, trimmed of excess fat
Sea salt and freshly ground black pepper
Lemon wedges, to serve

1. To prepare the cauliflower, either hold the stalk of the cauliflower and grate it on the large holes of a box grater, or break into florets and pulse briefly in a food processor until you get a rice-like consistency.

2. Put the cauliflower into a large serving bowl and drizzle with 1 tablespoon of the olive oil, then toss to coat.

3. Add the cherry tomatoes, red onion and cucumber to the bowl and mix. Roll the bunch of parsley up tightly into a cigar shape and finely shred the leaves until you reach the stalks. Discard the stalks, or save them for stock, and add the finely shredded leaves to the bowl. Finely shred the mint leaves and add them to the bowl.

4. Mix everything together well and squeeze over the juice of the lemon. Pour in the remaining olive oil and add a good pinch of salt and pepper. Mix well, taste and add a little more extra virgin olive oil or salt and pepper if needed.

5. Place a frying pan over a high heat and add a dash of rapeseed oil. When hot, add the lamb. Colour for 2½–3 minutes on each side until golden brown. Remove the meat from the pan and leave to rest.

6. Season the lamb with salt and pepper, then slice and serve with the tabbouleh and a wedge of lemon.

PER SERVING	
KCAL	391
FAT (g)	20.0
SATURATES (g)	5.0
CARBS (g)	11.0
SUGARS (g)	9.0
FIBRE (g)	6.0
PROTEIN (g)	38.0
SALT (g)	0.26

GOOD TO KNOW
As a chef, I am used to peeling and deseeding cucumbers, but given that the skin and seeds are packed with soluble fibre and other useful nutrients, it's worth keeping them intact here. Make sure you give them a good wash before eating, though.

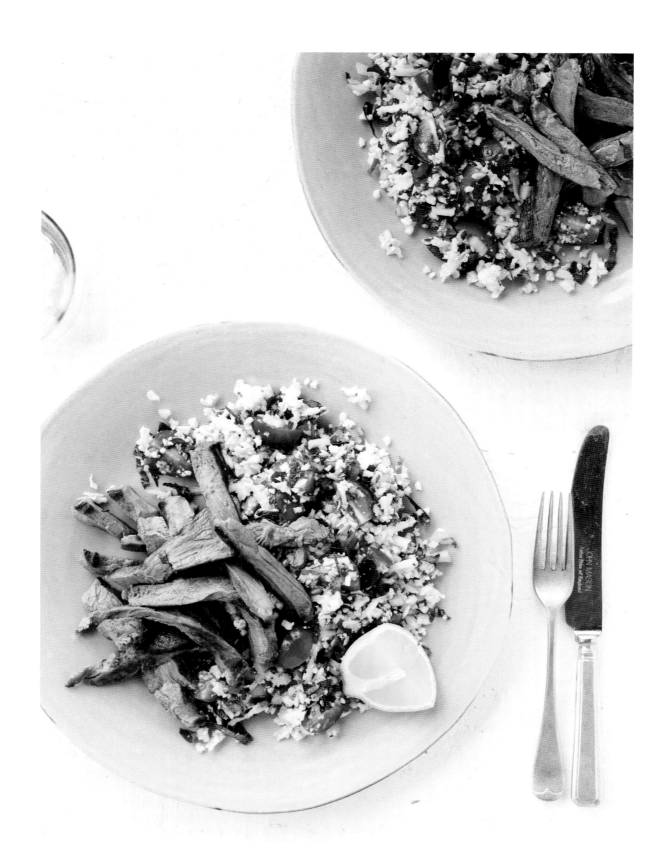

SEA BASS CEVICHE WITH TOMATO, LEMON AND CHILLI

SERVES 4

Ceviche (raw fish marinated in lemon or lime juice) is a brilliant dish to eat when trying to be healthy – it is naturally low in fat but punchy in flavour, and because the fish isn't exposed to heat, it retains all the goodness that might be damaged during cooking. Make sure to use the freshest fish you can find – it makes all the difference to the finished dish. This is also good made with scallops, sea bream or any other meaty white fish, and served with unsalted tortilla chips or toasted rye bread and a green salad.

400g sea bass fillets, skin removed, pin-boned and cut into bite-sized chunks
¼ red onion, peeled and very finely sliced
1 long red chilli, deseeded and finely chopped
Juice of 1½ lemons
4 medium, ripe tomatoes, finely diced
Small bunch of flat-leaf parsley, half the leaves picked, half finely chopped
Sea salt and freshly ground black pepper

1. Place the sea bass chunks, onion, chilli, lemon juice, half the tomatoes, the finely chopped parsley and a couple of pinches of salt in a large mixing bowl. Toss well to mix, then leave to stand for 10 minutes (or up to 30 minutes).

2. Once ready to serve, transfer the ceviche to a serving plate or shallow bowl and sprinkle over the remaining tomatoes and parsley leaves. Taste and adjust the seasoning as necessary, then serve immediately.

PER SERVING	
KCAL	191
FAT (g)	10.0
SATURATES (g)	2.0
CARBS (g)	4.0
SUGARS (g)	4.0
FIBRE (g)	1.0
PROTEIN (g)	21.0
SALT (g)	0.19

WHEN TO DRESS CEVICHE
Don't dress the ceviche until you are almost ready to eat it, otherwise the fish will 'cook' in the acid of the lemon juice and lose its firm texture. Ideally the fish should be left to marinate for just 10 minutes, and definitely no more than 30.

COURGETTE AND FENNEL CARPACCIO

SERVE 4 AS A SIDE

Finding new ways to include more vegetables, especially raw ones, in our diet can be challenging. Serving them in this way, very finely sliced and 'cooked' in a little lemon juice, is really simple, very refreshing and deceptively impressive – especially when garnished with jewel-like pomegranate seeds, fresh mint and black sesame seeds. It looks stunning! To make it a bit more substantial, crumble some feta or goat's cheese over the top.

1 large fennel bulb
Zest and juice of ½ lemon
2 medium courgettes
2 tbsp extra virgin olive oil
1 handful mint leaves, shredded
Seeds of ½ pomegranate
2 tsp black sesame seeds (optional)
Sea salt and freshly ground black pepper

1. Halve and finely slice the fennel bulb, using either a mandolin or a very sharp knife. Put the wafer-thin slices into a bowl and squeeze over the lemon juice.

2. Using a vegetable peeler, peel thin strips from the courgettes and add them to the bowl with the fennel.

3. Season the fennel and the courgettes generously with salt and pepper and drizzle with the olive oil. Toss to coat everything and leave to stand for 10 minutes.

4. After 10 minutes, toss through half the shredded mint leaves, taste and adjust the seasoning as necessary, adding more lemon juice if required, then arrange the salad on a serving plate. Scatter over the pomegranate seeds, lemon zest and the remaining shredded mint leaves and finish with a sprinkling of the black sesame seeds, if using.

PER SERVING	
KCAL	106
FAT (g)	6.0
SATURATES (g)	1.0
CARBS (g)	7.0
SUGARS (g)	6.0
FIBRE (g)	6.0
PROTEIN (g)	3.0
SALT (g)	0.04

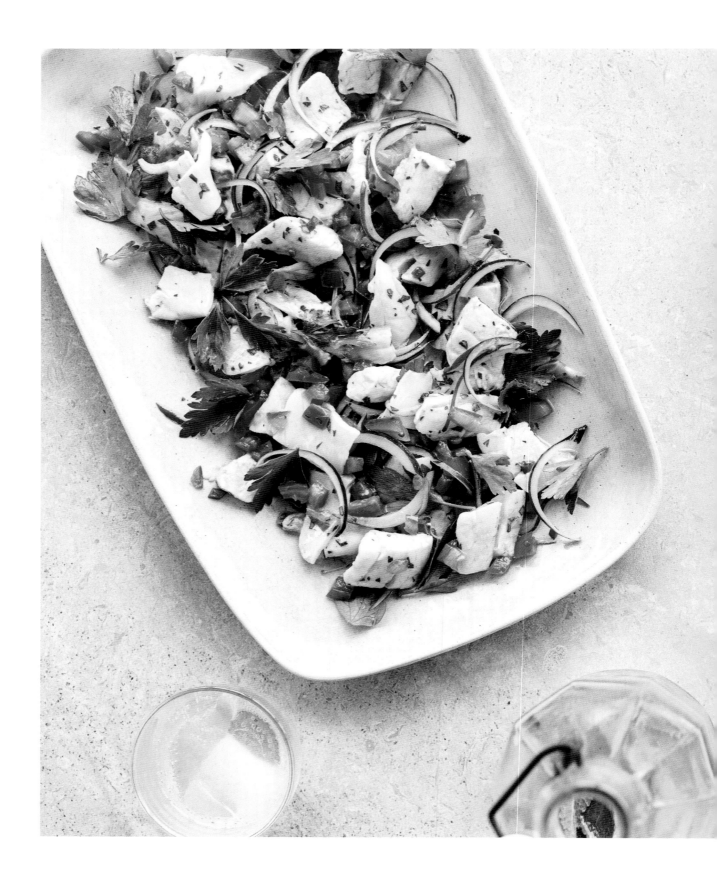

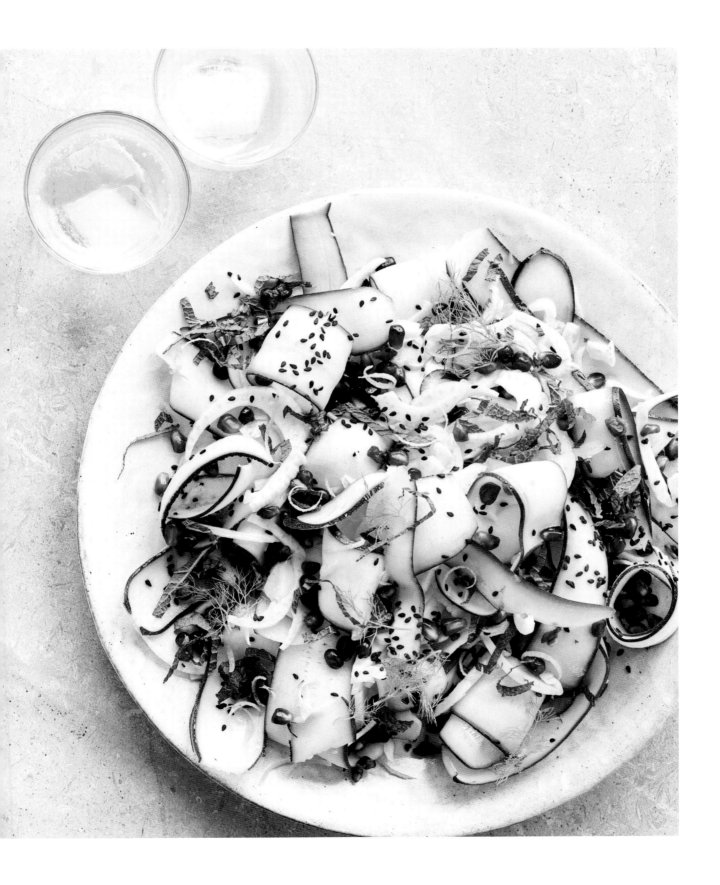

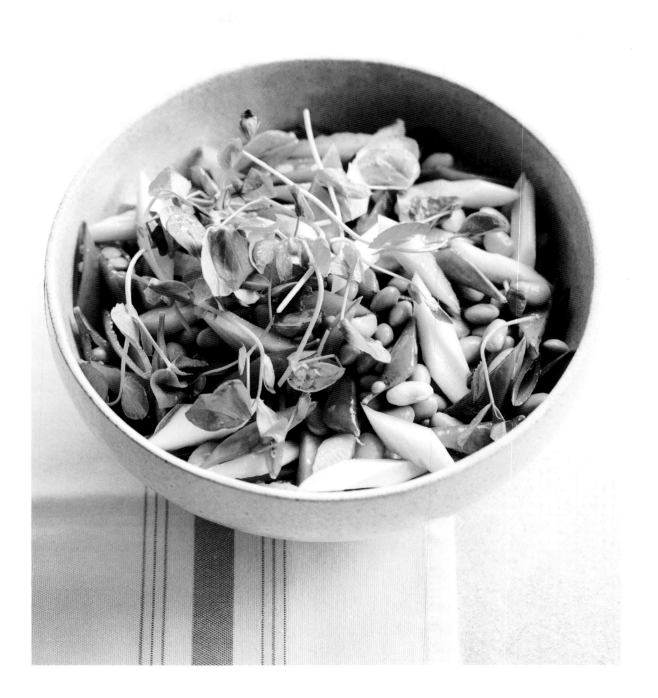

EDAMAME, SUGAR SNAP AND CELERY SALAD

SERVES 4 AS A SIDE

This is a brilliantly vibrant, green salad to add crunch to meat and fish dishes like the Miso Cod on page 64 or the Tuna Steak on page 67. You can buy edamame or soya beans in their pods or podded from most supermarkets these days but if you can't find fresh edamame, buy the frozen beans – like peas they are frozen within hours of being picked so they are still full of nutrients.

350g podded edamame beans (soya beans)
200g sugar snap peas, topped and tailed
3 celery sticks, trimmed, any leaves reserved
Pea shoots, to garnish

FOR THE DRESSING
1 tbsp rice vinegar
1 tbsp soy sauce
1 garlic clove, crushed
2 tbsp flavourless oil, e.g. groundnut

1. If the edamame beans need cooking, boil them in plenty of salted boiling water according to the packet instructions. Drain and run under the cold tap to cool or place in a bowl of iced water to prevent further cooking. Once cool, drain and pat dry.

2. Meanwhile, slice the sugar snaps diagonally into thirds and put them into a bowl.

3. Halve each celery stick lengthways and slice on the diagonal into 1cm wide pieces. Put them into the bowl with the sugar snap peas and the edamame beans.

4. Whisk together the ingredients for the dressing in a small bowl, then pour over the vegetables and toss well until everything is evenly coated. Serve immediately, garnished with the reserved celery leaves and pea shoots.

HOW TO DEFROST FROZEN EDAMAME BEANS
To defrost frozen edamame beans, put them in a microwaveable bowl with a tablespoon of water, cover and cook for 3 minutes or as per packet instructions, or blanch in a saucepan of boiling water for 3 minutes.

PER SERVING	
KCAL	182
FAT (g)	10.0
SATURATES (g)	2.0
CARBS (g)	8.0
SUGARS (g)	5.0
FIBRE (g)	6.0
PROTEIN (g)	12.0
SALT (g)	0.64

WHOLE BAKED TANDOORI-SPICED CAULIFLOWER

SERVES 6 AS A SIDE

Baking cauliflower whole in this way is so simple but it looks really impressive. Make it the centrepiece of an Indian banquet and cut it open at the table as though you were slicing a cake. It's as tasty as it looks and yet it's incredibly easy to cook – just remember to allow a bit of time for the spiced yoghurt marinade to really permeate the densely packed florets.

2 garlic cloves, peeled
2cm piece of fresh root ginger, peeled
1 tbsp tandoori masala spice mix
1 tsp chilli powder (optional)
Juice of ½ lemon
150g natural yoghurt
1 medium cauliflower, leaves removed and
   base trimmed flat
Olive oil
Dried chilli flakes, for serving (optional)
Sea salt

1. Using a fine grater such as a microplane, grate the garlic and ginger into a large mixing bowl. Add the tandoori masala, chilli powder (if using) and lemon juice and mix into a paste. Add the yoghurt and stir thoroughly. Season well with salt.

2. Place the cauliflower, base-side up, in the bowl. Using clean hands, spread the yoghurt marinade all over the cauliflower, then leave it to marinate for at least 20 minutes, or up to 12 hours (cover the bowl and put it into the fridge if marinating for longer than 20 minutes).

3. When ready to cook, preheat the oven to 180°C/ gas 4.

4. Put the cauliflower, base-side down, on a baking tray rubbed with a little olive oil and pour over any extra marinade still in the bowl. Put the tray into the preheated oven and bake for 35–40 minutes until golden and tender.

5. Put the cauliflower on a serving plate, sprinkle with chilli flakes, if using, and slice it into wedges like a cake to serve.

PER SERVING	
KCAL	66
FAT (g)	2.0
SATURATES (g)	1.0
CARBS (g)	6.0
SUGARS (g)	5.0
FIBRE (g)	2.0
PROTEIN (g)	4.0
SALT (g)	0.93

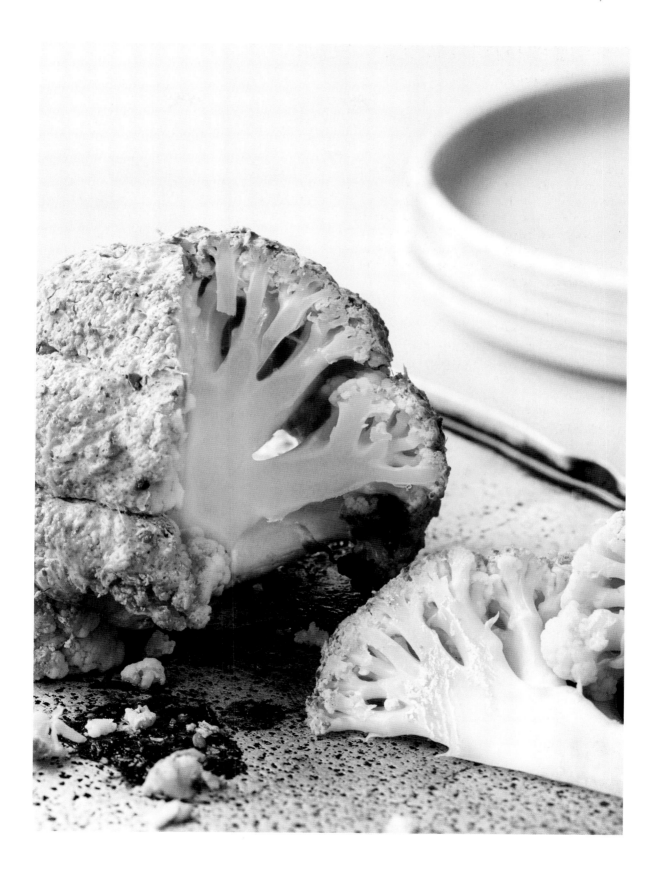

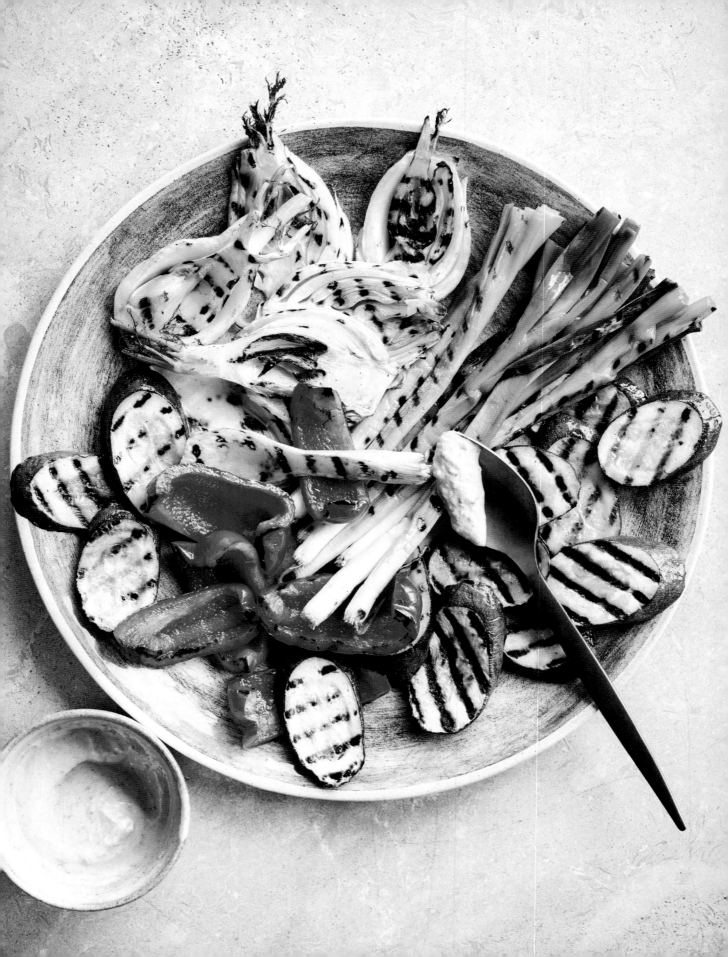

CHARGRILLED VEGETABLES WITH BAGNA CÀUDA DRESSING

SERVES 6 AS A STARTER OR SIDE

Bagna càuda roughly translates as 'hot bath' and refers to an intensely flavoured hot dip popular in the Piedmont region of Italy. It is also great cold and makes a delicious dressing for raw or chargrilled vegetables and salads to accompany grilled chicken, fish or lamb. This is a really good dish to make ahead because the flavours really intensify over time.

1 small fennel bulb, cut vertically into 1cm thick slices attached by the root
1 red pepper, deseeded and cut into approximately 6 large pieces
2 courgettes, trimmed and cut diagonally into 1cm thick slices
8 spring onions, trimmed
Olive oil, for drizzling

FOR THE BAGNA CÀUDA DRESSING
1 x 50g tin anchovies in extra virgin olive oil (oil reserved)
1 tbsp capers, drained and rinsed
2 garlic cloves, peeled and roughly chopped
Zest and juice of ½ lemon
50ml olive oil
Sea salt and freshly ground black pepper

1. To make the dressing, put the anchovies and their oil (apart from ½ a tablespoon), capers, garlic and lemon zest into a small food processor and blend until smooth.

2. Add the lemon juice with a pinch of pepper and mix together.

3. With the motor running, pour in the olive oil and about 3 tablespoons of cold water. Taste and adjust the seasoning if necessary.

4. Heat a griddle pan over a medium heat.

5. Put the vegetables into a bowl and drizzle with a little olive oil. Season with a pinch of salt and pepper and toss to make sure all the vegetables are coated.

6. When the griddle is hot, grill the vegetables in batches until they are all tender and lightly charred. Transfer to a serving platter once cooked.

7. Drizzle the bagna càuda dressing over the vegetables or serve it in a separate bowl for dipping.

PER SERVING	
KCAL	161
FAT (g)	14.0
SATURATES (g)	2.0
CARBS (g)	3.0
SUGARS (g)	3.0
FIBRE (g)	3.0
PROTEIN (g)	3.0
SALT (g)	0.85

SHAVED ASPARAGUS
AND HAZELNUT SALAD

SERVES 4 AS A SIDE

Shaving raw asparagus is such a good way to
serve the nation's favourite seasonal vegetable
and it makes a change from steaming or boiling it.
Plus it retains all its flavour, crunch and goodness.
The shavings make a great crisp salad that would
be a lovely summer starter or accompaniment to
grilled halloumi or creamy burrata.

50g blanched hazelnuts
3 tbsp hazelnut or walnut oil (if unavailable,
    use extra virgin olive oil)
Zest and juice of ½ lemon
1 tbsp white wine vinegar
500g thick asparagus spears
Sea salt and freshly ground black pepper

1. Toast the hazelnuts in a small, dry frying pan over
a medium heat until golden. Remove and roughly
chop, then leave to one side.

2. In a large mixing bowl, whisk together the hazelnut
oil, lemon juice, vinegar and a pinch of salt and
pepper until combined. Taste and adjust the seasoning
as needed.

3. Holding on to the woody end of the asparagus,
shave the spears into long thin strips with a vegetable
peeler or a very sharp knife. Put the shavings into the
bowl with the dressing and gently toss to coat.

4. Place the dressed asparagus on a serving plate or
in a bowl and scatter over the lemon zest and the
chopped hazelnuts. Serve immediately.

PER SERVING	
KCAL	196
FAT (g)	17.0
SATURATES (g)	1.0
CARBS (g)	3.0
SUGARS (g)	3.0
FIBRE (g)	4.0
PROTEIN (g)	6.0
SALT (g)	0.01

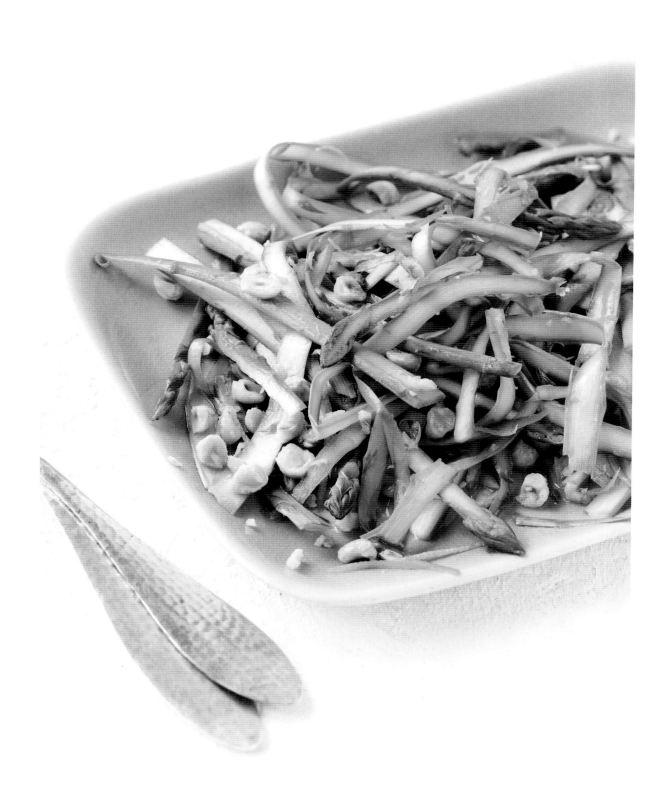

HEALTHY SNACKS AND NOT-TOO-SWEET TREATS

CUCUMBER AND MINT LEMONADE

SERVES 4

Homemade lemonade bears very little resemblance to the commercially produced stuff; it is less sweet and cloying and therefore much more refreshing on a hot summer's day. Adding the cucumber and mint makes it even more delicious and adds an extra handful of vitamins and minerals, making it the perfect way to keep everyone hydrated.

125ml lemon juice (from approximately 2–3 lemons)
2 cucumbers, sliced
5–6 mint sprigs, leaves removed, plus extra to garnish
1–3 tbsp agave syrup, to taste
Soda water
Lemon slices, to serve

1. Put the lemon juice, sliced cucumbers and mint leaves into a blender and blitz until smooth, adding a little water if necessary. Once smooth, pour the liquid through a sieve or muslin into a large jug, pressing the pulp with the back of a clean spoon to get as much liquid out as possible.

2. Taste the liquid and sweeten as necessary, stirring in the agave syrup a little at a time. Add a couple of handfuls of ice and top up with very cold soda water until the desired dilution is reached (aim for roughly 1 part lemonade to 1 part water).

3. Serve chilled, with lots of ice, a slice of lemon and a sprig of mint in each glass.

PER SERVING	
KCAL	46
FAT (g)	1.0
SATURATES (g)	0.0
CARBS (g)	6.0
SUGARS (g)	6.0
FIBRE (g)	1.0
PROTEIN (g)	2.0
SALT (g)	0.02

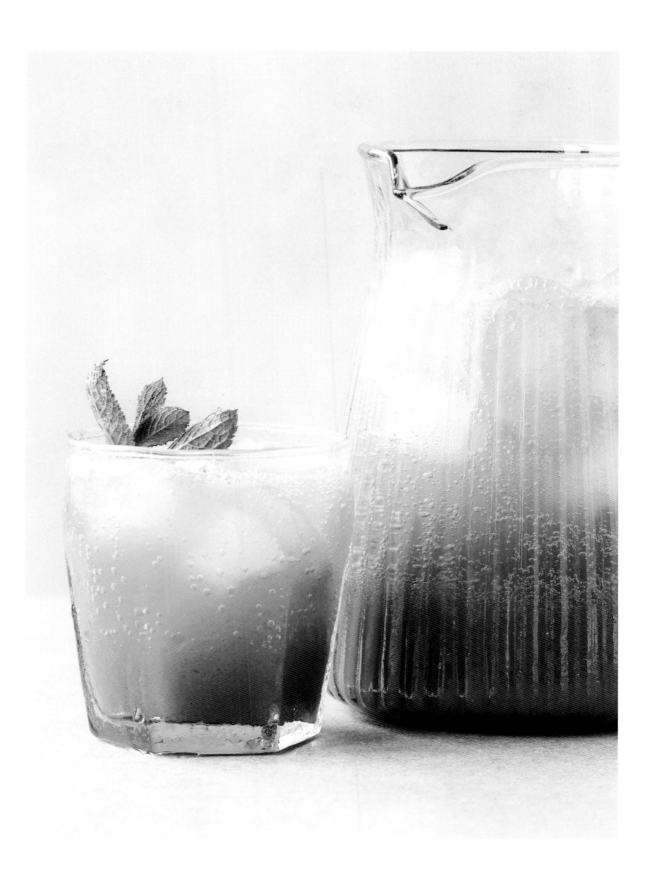

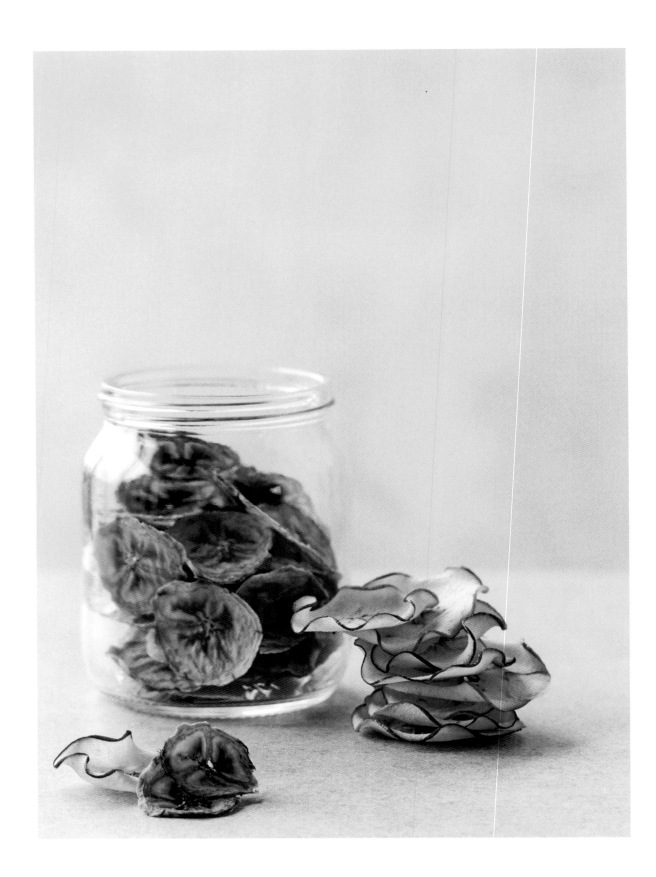

BANANA AND APPLE CRISPS

SERVES 4

These healthy crisps will provide both the sweetness and the crunch that we often crave when we're trying to eat more healthily and reduce our sugar intake. They make a great snack for kids, who end up eating lots of fruit without really realizing it. Great for adults too, so make a big batch and keep them in an airtight container to last the week. These crisps are also very low in fat, so add them to the list of guilt-free snacks on page 169 if you are watching your weight.

2 apples
2 bananas, peeled

1. Preheat the oven to 90°C/gas ¼.

2. Line 2–3 large baking trays with greaseproof paper.

3. Slice the apples and bananas very finely with a mandolin or sharp knife and lay the slices on the lined baking trays in a single layer.

4. Put the trays into the preheated oven and bake for 1½–2 hours. The apples will be crisp before the bananas, so check them after 1½ hours. The bananas can take up to half an hour longer in the oven, depending on their thickness.

5. Leave the fruit crisps to cool on the tray, then transfer to an airtight container and eat within 1 week.

VARIATIONS
This method also works really well for pineapple, pears and star fruit, and you can try sprinkling the fruit with spices like cinnamon or cardamom for even more flavour.

PER SERVING	
KCAL	70
FAT (g)	0.3
SATURATES (g)	0.1
CARBS (g)	15.0
SUGARS (g)	14.0
FIBRE (g)	1.0
PROTEIN (g)	1.0
SALT (g)	0.0

SMOKY FLAGEOLET BEAN HOUMOUS

SERVES 4

Living in California for part of the year means my family and I have all developed a deep love of Mexican food. I find the smoky, hot flavours are creeping into familiar family dishes more and more, like in this flageolet houmous which is seasoned with a very Mexican combination of chipotle chilli paste, cumin, lime and coriander. It's now a favourite snack wherever we are.

Olive oil
1 small onion, peeled and diced
2 garlic cloves, peeled and roughly chopped
2 tsp cumin seeds
1 x 400g tin flageolet beans (if unavailable, replace with cannellini or other white beans), drained and rinsed
1–1½ tsp chipotle paste, to taste
Zest and juice of 1 lime
Small bunch of coriander, roughly chopped
Sea salt and freshly ground black pepper

1. Heat a small frying pan over a medium heat and add a dash of oil. Once hot, sauté the diced onion with a pinch of salt for 5–6 minutes, until softened.

2. Add the garlic and cumin seeds and continue to cook for 1–2 minutes, until the garlic has softened and the cumin is fragrant. Remove the pan from the heat and transfer to the bowl of a food processor.

3. Add the beans, chipotle paste (starting with 1 teaspoon), a drizzle of olive oil (about ½ tablespoon) and the lime zest to the bowl and blitz until smooth. Taste and add a little more chipotle paste if you like it spicy.

4. Add half the lime juice and the chopped coriander and blitz again until smooth with flecks of green. Taste and add a little more lime juice, salt and pepper if necessary. Serve immediately, or store covered in the fridge for up to 3 days.

PER SERVING	
KCAL	80
FAT (g)	3.0
SATURATES (g)	0.3
CARBS (g)	8.0
SUGARS (g)	1.0
FIBRE (g)	3.0
PROTEIN (g)	4.0
SALT (g)	0.09

VARIATION
Chipotle paste is available online or from most supermarkets. If you can't find it, replace it with 1–2 teaspoons of smoked paprika, stirring it in with the cumin.

MINTED BABA GANOUSH

SERVES 4

Aubergines are one of my favourite vegetables; they're so full of flavour, and making a creamy, smoky dip out of the flesh is a really good way of showcasing them. Serve this as a snack with crudités or Pitta Crisps (see page 266) or as a side with grilled meats like sausages, lamb and duck. The flavour of any dish made with aubergines improves over time, so this can easily be made two or three days ahead and will be more delicious for it.

2 medium aubergines
1 garlic clove, peeled and roughly chopped
1 tbsp tahini
6 mint sprigs, leaves finely chopped
Juice of 1–2 lemons, to taste
Sea salt and freshly ground black pepper

TO GARNISH
Seeds from ½ pomegranate
2 mint sprigs, leaves shredded

1. Turn on two rings of your gas hob. Place an aubergine directly over each ring, turning regularly until the flesh is soft and the skin is charred all over. Leave to cool.

2. Slice the aubergines in half and scoop out the flesh with a spoon. Put the flesh into a food processor and blend until as smooth as possible.

3. Add the garlic, tahini, mint leaves and the juice of 1 lemon and season with salt and pepper. Blend again and taste to check the seasoning, adding more lemon juice if needed.

4. Serve the baba ganoush in a bowl with the pomegranate seeds and shredded mint leaves sprinkled over the top.

HOW TO CHAR AUBERGINES
Lining your hob with kitchen foil before charring the aubergines will make clearing up much quicker and easier. If you don't have a gas hob, cook the aubergines in an oven preheated to 200°C/gas 6 for 35–45 minutes, or turn them frequently under a hot grill until really soft inside and blackened on the outside.

PER SERVING	
KCAL	87
FAT (g)	3.0
SATURATES (g)	1.0
CARBS (g)	8.0
SUGARS (g)	7.0
FIBRE (g)	7.0
PROTEIN (g)	3.0
SALT (g)	0.01

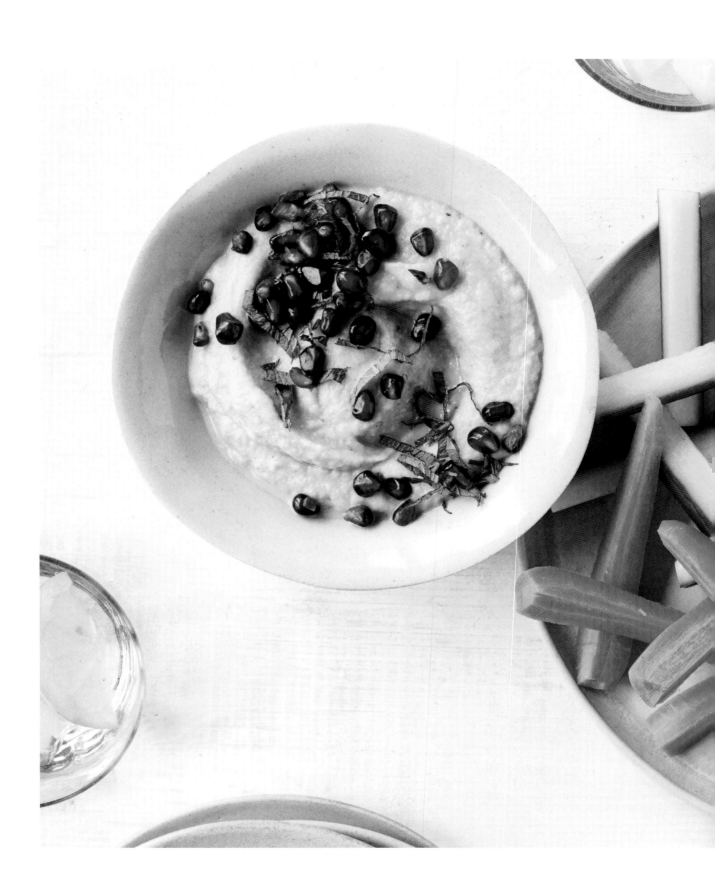

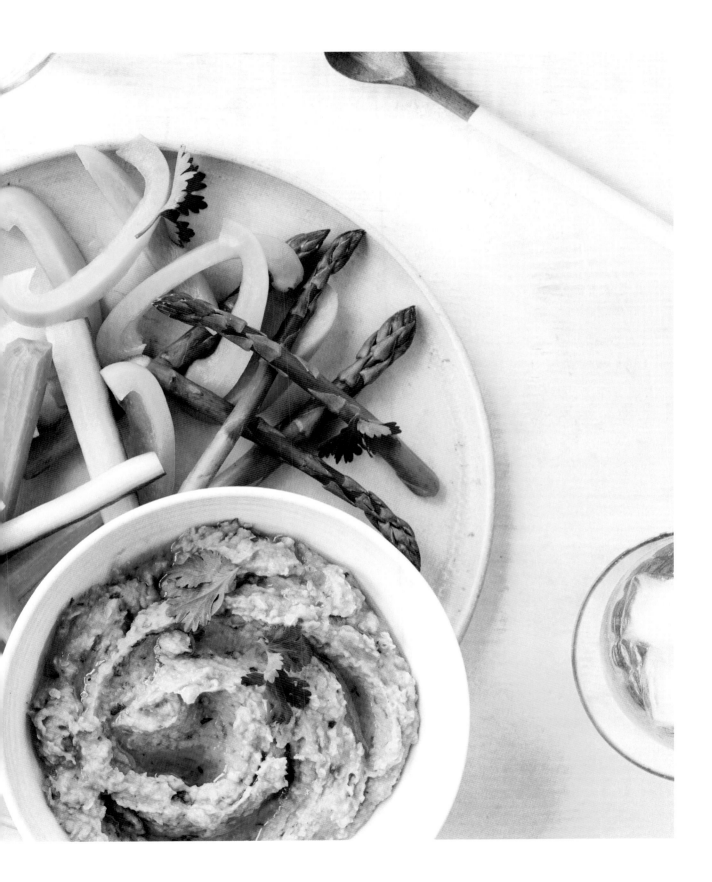

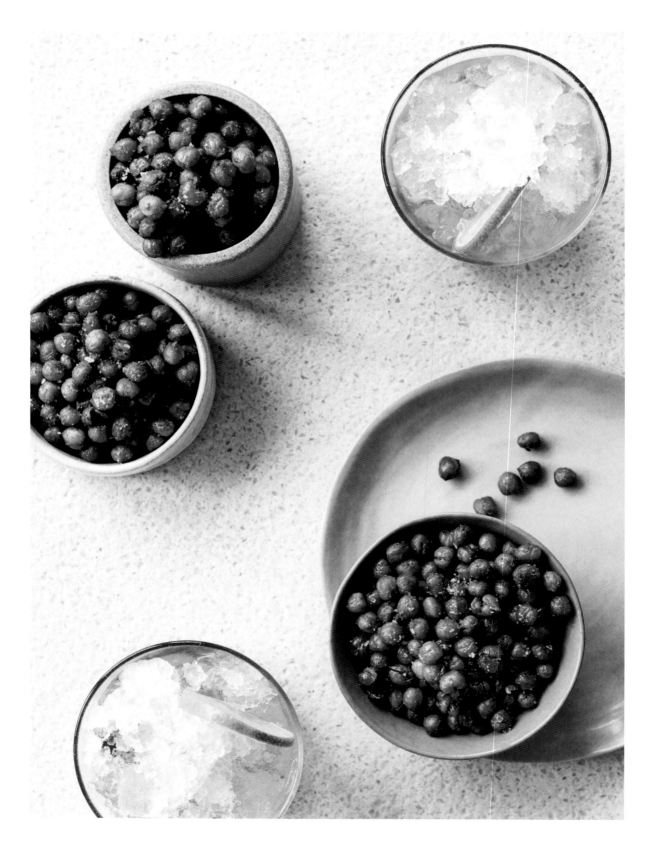

CRUNCHY CHICKPEAS

SERVES 4

It's rare to find a satisfying savoury snack to replace crisps, but these chickpeas are just that – salty, spicy and moreish, they really hit the spot with an evening drink or in front of a film. Double up the recipe for a crowd, as they are likely to disappear in seconds. Crunchy chickpeas are also a really healthy addition to salads and scattered on top of soups instead of croutons. Change the spices depending on your dish, or just season with salt and pepper.

2 x 400g tins chickpeas, drained, rinsed and dried very well
2 tbsp olive oil
2 tsp ground cumin
1 tsp cayenne pepper (optional)
Sea salt and freshly ground black pepper

1. Preheat the oven to 170°C/gas 3.

2. Make sure the chickpeas are completely dry, then spread them over two baking trays. Drizzle with the oil and sprinkle over the cumin and cayenne pepper, if using, then season with salt and pepper.

3. Put the trays into the preheated oven and roast for 15–20 minutes, or until the chickpeas are completely crisp. Check them after 10 minutes and give the tray a shake to move the chickpeas around.

4. Remove the trays from the oven and allow the chickpeas to cool before serving. Store in an airtight container for up to 3 days.

HOW TO MAKE THE CHICKPEAS CRISP UP
The trick to getting the chickpeas really crisp is to make sure they are as dry as possible before you put them into the oven.

PER SERVING	
KCAL	209
FAT (g)	9.0
SATURATES (g)	1.0
CARBS (g)	19.0
SUGARS (g)	1.0
FIBRE (g)	7.0
PROTEIN (g)	9.0
SALT (g)	0.01

CHARGRILLED PEACHES WITH GRANOLA CRUMBLE

SERVES 4

This is a wonderfully summery pudding that is one of my daughter Tilly's favourites. It's a really simple, light dessert with a satisfying crunch and is the perfect way to end a summer lunch or barbecue. When peaches are out of season, you can replace them with ripe pears. The nutty granola crumble is also delicious sprinkled over yoghurt or ice cream – it will last up to ten days in an airtight container.

4 semi-ripe peaches or nectarines, halved
   and stoned
Melted coconut oil or flavourless oil,
   e.g. groundnut, for brushing

FOR THE CRUMBLE
30g rolled oats
1 tbsp maple syrup
1 tbsp coconut oil or ½ tbsp flavourless oil,
   e.g. groundnut
25g almonds, roughly chopped
25g pecans, roughly chopped
Pinch of sea salt
0% fat Greek yoghurt, to serve (optional)

1. Preheat the oven to 180°C/gas 4.

2. To make the crumble, mix together the oats, maple syrup and coconut oil (melted if necessary) until the oats are completely coated. Add the chopped nuts and a pinch of salt and mix again.

3. Pour the oats and nuts on to a baking tray and put this into the preheated oven for 7–10 minutes, until the oats are golden and crunchy.

4. Meanwhile, heat a griddle pan over a medium-high heat. Brush the cut sides of the peaches with a little oil and place on the hot griddle, cut side down. Leave on the griddle without disturbing for 3 minutes to allow the griddle marks to develop.

5. Turn over and cook for a further 2 minutes on the other side.

6. Serve the peaches warm, sprinkled with the nutty crumble. Serve with 0% fat Greek yoghurt, if you like.

PER SERVING	
KCAL	207
FAT (g)	13.0
SATURATES (g)	4.0
CARBS (g)	17.0
SUGARS (g)	11.0
FIBRE (g)	3.0
PROTEIN (g)	4.0
SALT (g)	0.13

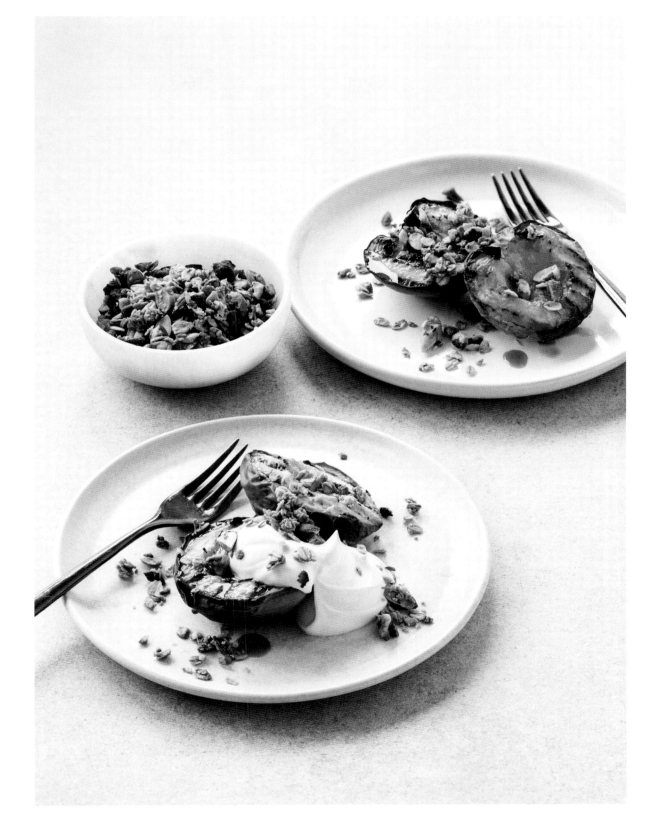

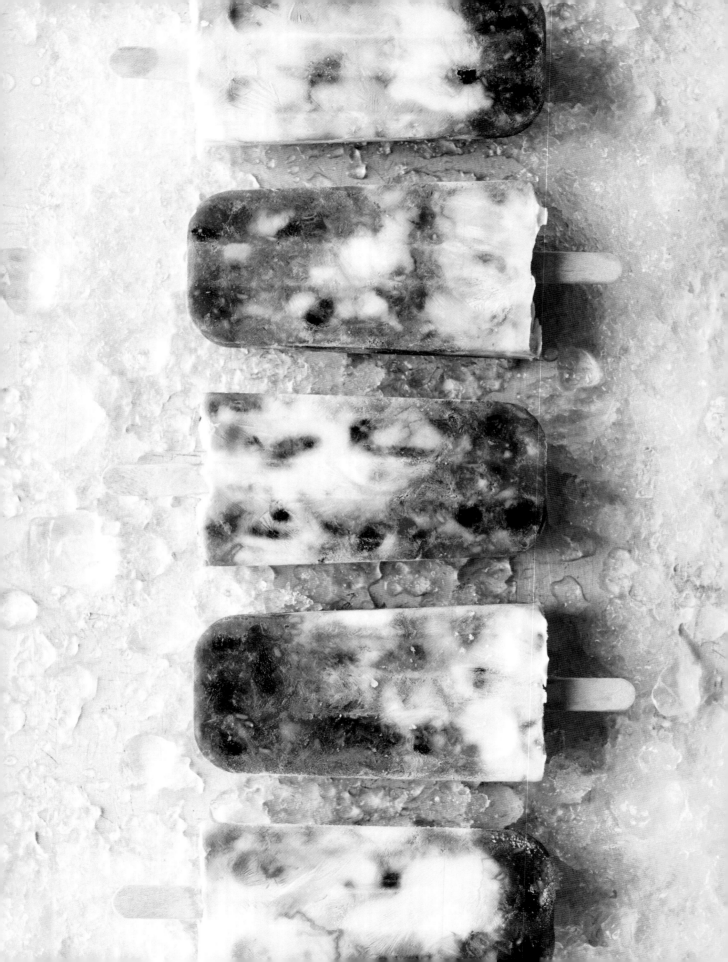

YOGHURT AND BERRY ICE LOLLIES

MAKES 6 LOLLIES

This versatile recipe is a great way to get kids to eat more fruit in summer and to avoid commercially made high-sugar lollies and ice creams. Experiment with the flavour of the yoghurt and swap the berries for diced banana, kiwi, mango or melon, depending on what you have in your fruit bowl, but remember they take at least four hours to freeze solid.

100g fresh or frozen berries, such as strawberries, raspberries or blackcurrants (defrosted if frozen), roughly chopped
1½ tbsp runny honey
250g 0% fat Greek yoghurt

1. Mash together the berries and half the honey with a fork until roughly puréed.

2. Put the yoghurt into a bowl and mix in the remaining honey.

3. Spoon the mashed berries into the bottom of lolly moulds, then spoon the yoghurt on top gently, mixing it together to create a ripple effect.

4. Put in the lolly sticks and place in the freezer for at least 4 hours, or overnight.

5. To serve, remove from the freezer and allow to warm slightly or hold under warm running water before trying to pull the lollies out of the moulds.

GOOD TO KNOW
These ice lollies are low in fat and calories, so can still be indulged in if you are trying to lose weight.

PER SERVING	
KCAL	45
FAT (g)	0.0
SATURATES (g)	0.0
CARBS (g)	7.0
SUGARS (g)	7.0
FIBRE (g)	0.3
PROTEIN (g)	4.0
SALT (g)	0.14

CHOCOLATE AND AVOCADO MOUSSE

SERVES 8

If you like a hit of sweet at the end of a meal, try this knockout chocolate mousse. It's made with avocado, which may sound strange, but it has a silky, creamy texture which really works with the chocolate. The result is a surprisingly decadent pudding that is so much better for you than the egg-based classic. And if you think people will turn their noses up when they hear about the avocado, don't tell them until they've finished it – they'll never guess!

2 large ripe avocados, peeled and stoned
3–4 tbsp runny honey, to taste
1 tsp vanilla extract
50g raw cacao powder

1. Put the avocados into a food processor and blend until smooth.

2. Add 3 tablespoons of the honey with the vanilla and cacao powder and blend again until completely combined. Taste and add more honey if necessary.

3. Spoon the mousse into 8 shot or sweet wine glasses and put them into the fridge for an hour before serving.

PER SERVING	
KCAL	147
FAT (g)	10.0
SATURATES (g)	2.0
CARBS (g)	10.0
SUGARS (g)	6.0
FIBRE (g)	2.0
PROTEIN (g)	3.0
SALT (g)	0.02

HOW TO MEASURE HONEY
Because honey is so sticky, it can be difficult to measure it accurately – so much can be left behind on the spoon! If, however, you coat the measuring spoon with a thin layer of flavourless oil like groundnut, it will slip right off, ensuring that the right amount of honey makes it into your cooking.

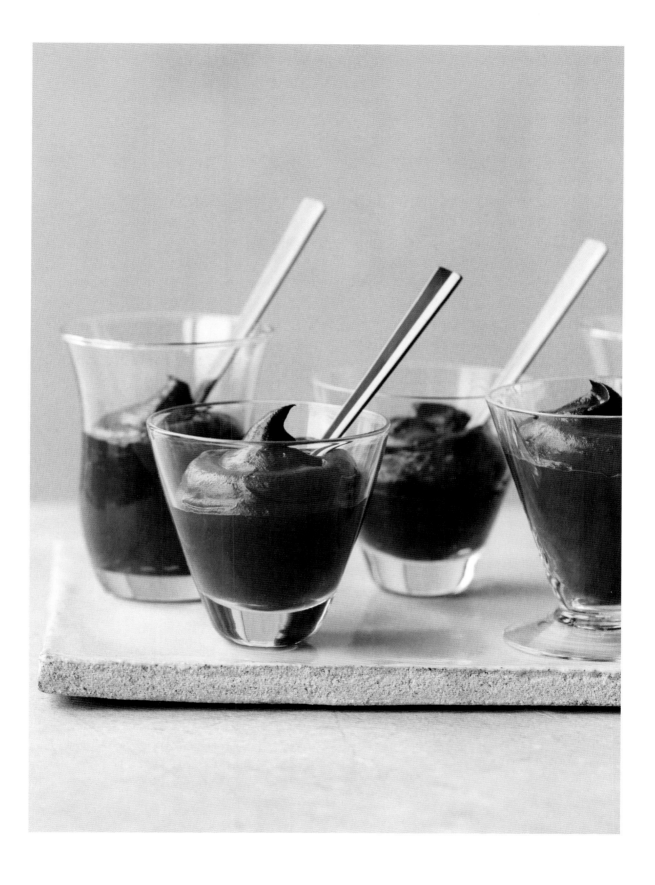

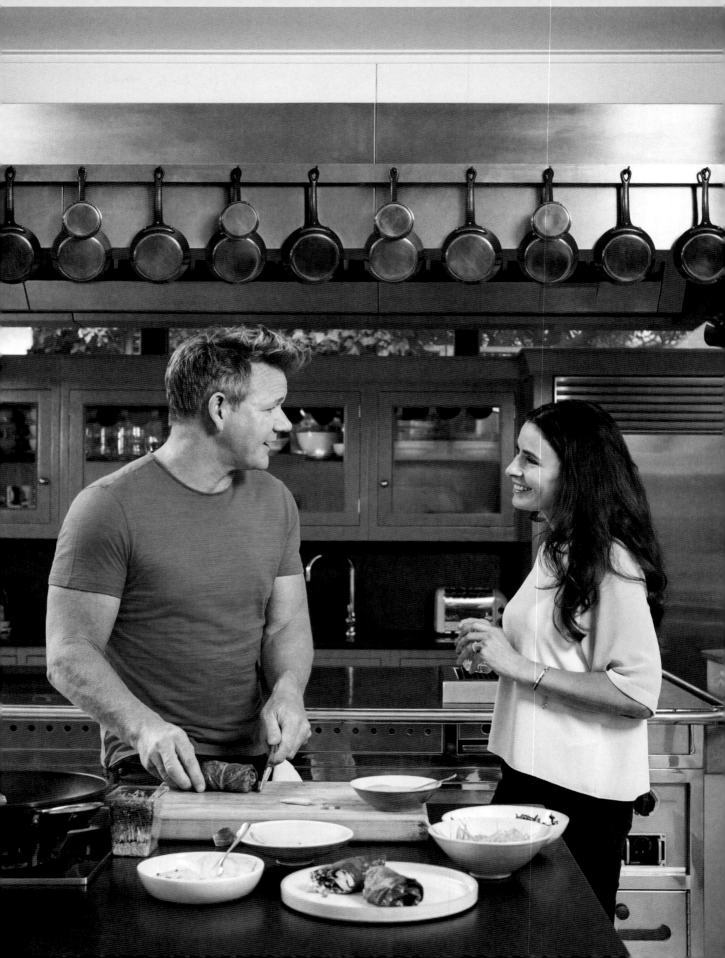

START-AS-YOU-MEAN-
TO-GO-ON BREAKFASTS

LIGHT LUNCHES TO
KEEP YOU ON TRACK

LEAN SUPPERS AND SIDES

GUILT-FREE TREATS

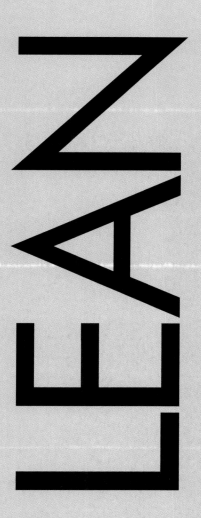

THOUGH I HAVE LOST WEIGHT IN MY TIME, I HAVE NEVER REALLY BEEN ON A FORMAL DIET.

Maybe it's because I'm a chef, but I hate the idea of having to eat less or cutting out food groups or going hungry. Instead, I eat more carefully. I choose dishes and ways of cooking that are naturally low in fat and calories but big on flavour and satisfaction. I give favourite dishes a lean makeover and make sure I stock up on low-fat snacks. The trick for me is to not feel deprived and to enjoy the food I eat as much as I usually do. That, and to make sure I am getting plenty of exercise to burn up the food that I am consuming.

Essentially, the weight loss equation is really very simple. To lose weight, the energy generated by what you eat needs to be less than the amount of energy you are burning up through activity. If you are consuming more food than you are using, your body will lay down the excess as body fat. If you consume less than you need to, your body will use up this stored energy and you will lose weight.

Unfortunately, most adults consume more calories than they need and while some people can get away with it, many of us are carrying around extra weight as a result. The simple solution is to eat less and start doing more exercise, but as that can sound a bit daunting, lots of people fail or don't even try. Personally, I like to think of it not as eating less but as eating better and getting more active, so that you can still eat many of the foods that you love.

Increasing activity levels will help you to lose weight faster, not simply because this burns up stored body fat but also because it increases your metabolism and, by replacing fat with muscle, you burn more calories while resting. But you don't have to start running ultramarathons – unless you want to, of course! Getting active can start with getting off the bus earlier than you need to, dancing around the kitchen, doing some gardening or signing up for a charity run. The fitter you get, the easier exercise becomes and the more weight you will lose.

I'm not saying it's easy. It involves willpower and determination and it won't happen overnight. The trick is to have manageable goals. When I needed to tackle my own weight gain, I didn't immediately sign up for an Ironman triathlon; I started running 5km at the gym, then 10km, and it went from there. When Tana was getting back into shape after our four children were born, she always had a pair of jeans that she wanted to get back into. The thought of being able to fit into those trousers kept her going when it was tough.

This section is full of lean but satisfying dishes that we rely on at home to keep us on track. For me, the important thing is that they don't feel like diet food and I never feel like I'm depriving myself. There are sustaining salads, wraps and soups, flavours from Japan, Vietnam and North Africa, and even treats that are virtually guilt-free. It isn't easy but this is a great place to start.

ABOUT CALORIES

Personally, I have never counted calories. As a chef tasting lots of small mouthfuls all day, it would be impossible to add them all up! And I'm not necessarily suggesting that you count calories either, but it is a very useful way of judging food in terms of the all-important weight loss equation – i.e. the amount of energy consumed should be less than the amount used. Calories provide us with a clear numerical way of looking at food that can help to make this equation really straightforward.

Calories are basically a unit used to measure the amount of energy in food, and human beings need a certain number of calories per day to function. As a guide, an average man needs around 2,500 calories a day and an average woman needs around 2,000. As discussed, if you regularly consume more calories than this (and are only moderately active), over time you are likely to put on weight. If you are trying to lose weight, it is recommended that you reduce your daily allowance by 500 calories, to 2,000 calories per day if you are a man and 1,500 calories per day if you are a woman.

The calories in food come from macronutrients (carbohydrates, protein, fat), but each different macronutrient provides different amounts of calories per gram. Each gram of carbohydrate and protein provides 4 calories, while each gram of fat provides 9 calories. So you would have to eat more carbohydrates or protein to generate as many calories as fat. Or, putting it another way, cutting down on fat means you are consuming fewer calories more easily. The recipes in this section are generally lower in fat and sugar, to help you reduce your calorie intake by 500 calories a day, and they also include plenty of complex carbohydrates and lean proteins, to make you feel full and satiated and to keep you going in between meals.

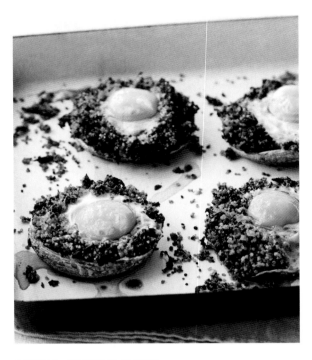

A WORD ABOUT ALCOHOL

Recent studies have shown that drinking alcohol in moderation may actually be good for your health. Apparently up to three to five drinks a week may help prevent heart attacks and increase life expectancy, which, if it turns out to be true, could be great news for those of us who like a glass of wine now and again. The bad news is that alcohol contains 7 calories per gram, which is almost as much as fat, and that doesn't include the sugary mixers that often come with it. To put this into context, drinking five pints of lager a week is the equivalent of eating 221 doughnuts in a year! Plus, these are known as 'empty calories' because they have no nutritional value whatsoever. On top of this, alcohol slows down the metabolism as the body prioritizes processing the booze rather than digesting food and burning energy.

So, if you are trying to lose weight, cutting back on alcohol is a really good way to keep your calorie intake down and your metabolism fired up. It's also much easier to stay on track if you don't drink; your resolve is immediately weakened by even one glass of wine or beer, and the food choices you make while drinking are often terrible – kebab, anyone? Then there's the hangover to contend with . . . If you really want to shift a few pounds, a dry period can help.

EATING OUT

When I was working in the kitchen full-time, I obviously didn't get to eat in restaurants very often, but these days I have more evenings off and I love going out for meals with my family to celebrate special occasions or just to check out new chefs and dishes. The trouble is that I know only too well that chefs don't hold back when it comes to the fattening stuff like butter, cream, cheese, sugar and chocolate. I don't want to feel deprived at home, let alone when I am out for dinner, so I set myself some rules which mean I can enjoy myself as much as everyone else. What follows is my advice for eating out when you are trying to stay slim.

Being starving hungry when you arrive at the table is a really bad idea, because you make terrible choices when you look at the menu and then tuck into the bread and butter, consuming half your allowed calories before the food even arrives! To avoid this, make sure you have a protein-rich lunch and a light afternoon snack to help you keep focused. If you don't want to eat anything beforehand, a clever trick is to look at the menu online, preferably when you aren't hungry, pick out the healthiest option and don't even look at the menu when you get there.

I've already covered alcohol, but just say no to a sugary aperitif or cocktail before you eat and restrict yourself to one glass of excellent wine or a favourite beer to be enjoyed with the food. Getting tipsy on an empty stomach will definitely lead to bad choices and more alcohol will add a lot of empty calories to an already indulgent meal. Say no to bread too. Yes, it's really delicious but as I have already said, you can consume lots of calories before your food has even arrived, and why pay to fill yourself up on something you can toast at home? You're there for the chef's expertise, so save your calories.

When we eat out as a family, everyone always wants three courses, so Tana and I share a starter and dessert, which keeps our overall intake down. If you aren't very good at sharing, choose a starter or a pudding rather than having both, or choose a second starter for your main course. If you can't resist something sweet at the end of a meal, order a cup of peppermint tea with a little honey stirred in, or have a square of dark chocolate on the way home. But if things go wrong and you just can't resist that chocolate mousse, go for an extra long run the next day as penance!

START-AS-YOU-MEAN-TO-GO-ON BREAKFASTS

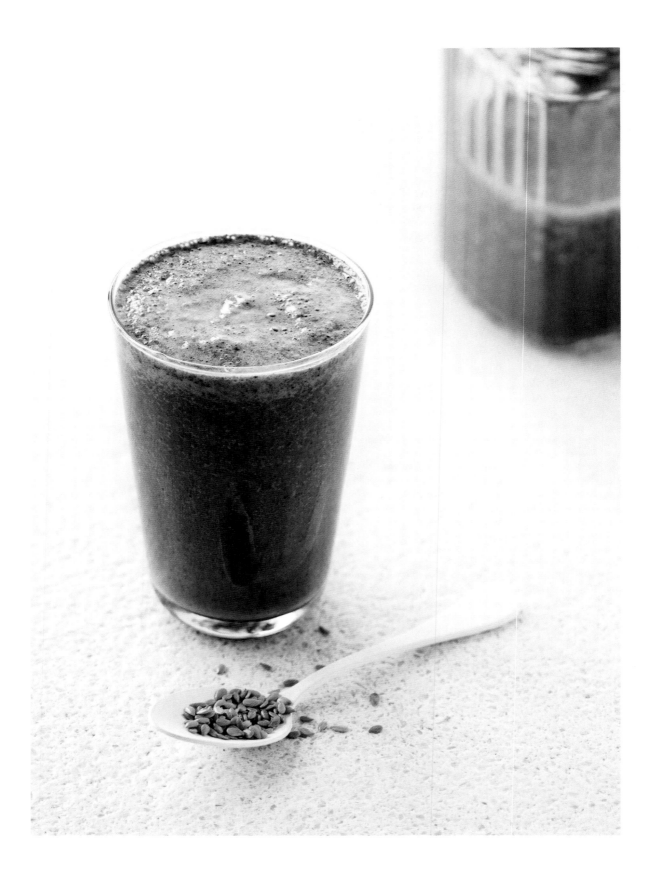

BERRY AND OAT SMOOTHIE

SERVES 1

Adding oats and flaxseeds to a fruit smoothie will not only help you feel fuller for longer but will also slow down the rate at which the natural sugars from the fruit hit your system, helping to avoid peaks and troughs in blood sugar levels for the rest of the day. You can also add other fruits such as strawberries, raspberries, pear, banana or mango, depending on what you have in the fruit bowl.

25g rolled oats
150ml semi-skimmed milk
2 tsp honey
75g blueberries
75g blackberries
2 tsp ground flaxseeds

1. Put the oats into a blender and pour over the milk. Leave to sit for 5 minutes.

2. Add the honey, blueberries, blackberries and ground flaxseeds and blitz until smooth.

GOOD TO KNOW
This would be a good pre-race or workout smoothie too.

PER SERVING	
KCAL	297
FAT (g)	8.0
SATURATES (g)	2.0
CARBS (g)	41.0
SUGARS (g)	24.0
FIBRE (g)	9.0
PROTEIN (g)	11.0
SALT (g)	0.18

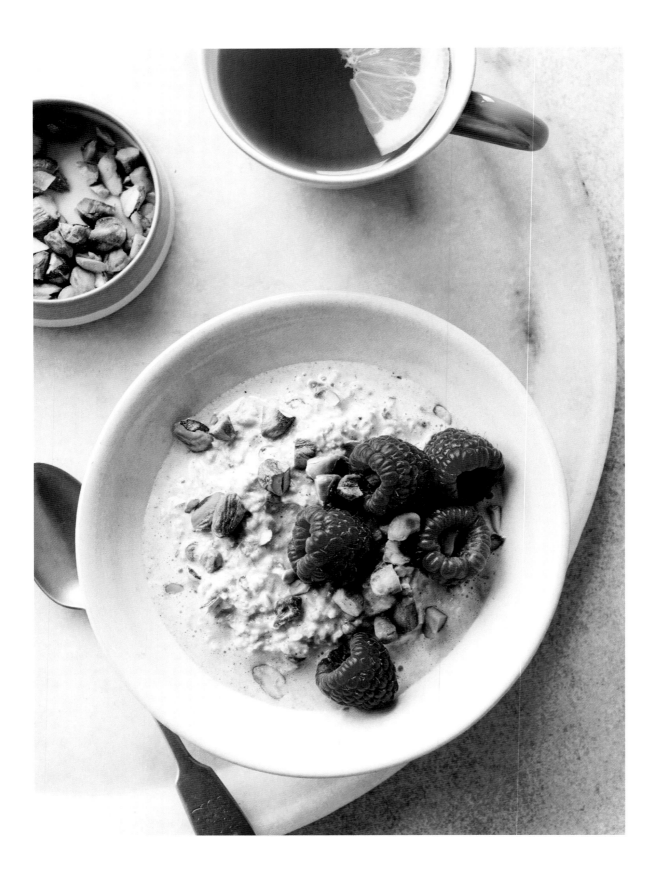

RASPBERRY AND HONEY OVERNIGHT OATS

SERVES 2

Preparing your breakfast the night before is a clever way to help you make a sensible decision when you're hungry first thing in the morning. You just open the fridge and tuck into the goodness of oats, honey and raspberries all ready to go. This is particularly good with a handful of chopped pistachio nuts sprinkled over the top, but leave them out if you are being very strict with yourself.

100g porridge oats
1 tsp mixed spice
200ml semi-skimmed milk
75g raspberries, plus a few extra to serve
25g honey
20g pistachio nuts, roughly chopped,
   to serve (optional)

1. Put the porridge oats into a large bowl and sprinkle over the mixed spice. Pour in the milk and mix together well.

2. In a separate bowl, crush the raspberries and honey together with the back of a fork until roughly mashed.

3. Stir the raspberry mixture through the oats, then divide between two bowls or airtight containers, cover and leave in the fridge overnight.

4. When ready to eat, remove the bowls from the fridge and top with a few extra raspberries and a sprinkle of chopped pistachios, if using.

PER SERVING	
KCAL	299
FAT (g)	6.0
SATURATES (g)	2.0
CARBS (g)	48.0
SUGARS (g)	15.0
FIBRE (g)	5.0
PROTEIN (g)	10.0
SALT (g)	0.16

SPINACH, TOMATO AND FETA SCRAMBLED EGGS

SERVES 4

Adding extra ingredients to scrambled eggs is really popular in the States, and I love this combination when I'm in LA. Feta is naturally lower in fat than many cheeses, and because the flavour is salty and intense, a little goes a long way. It also helps to keep the texture soft, as the eggs are less likely to overcook. These eggs are particularly good served with a little chilli sauce. For active days, serve the scrambled eggs on wholemeal or rye toast or with brown rice or quinoa, to make this a good breakfast for a training or race day.

Olive oil, for frying
12 cherry tomatoes, halved
100g spinach leaves, washed and dried
8 eggs
100g feta cheese, crumbled
Sea salt and freshly ground black pepper

1. Place a large, deep frying pan over a medium heat and add a dash of oil. Once hot, put the tomatoes, cut side down, into the pan and season with salt and pepper. Cook for 3–4 minutes, until they start to colour and caramelize slightly.

2. Turn the tomatoes over gently and put the spinach leaves on top. Cook for a further 3 minutes, then stir gently to mix the spinach and tomatoes together.

3. Meanwhile, crack the eggs into a bowl, season with a pinch of pepper and beat to combine.

4. Once the spinach has wilted, reduce the heat to medium-low, pour in the eggs and add the crumbled feta. Gently cook, stirring regularly, until the eggs are mixed with the other ingredients and scrambled but not set.

5. Remove the pan from the heat, check the seasoning, and serve immediately.

PER SERVING	
KCAL	239
FAT (g)	16.0
SATURATES (g)	6.0
CARBS (g)	2.0
SUGARS (g)	2.0
FIBRE (g)	1.0
PROTEIN (g)	19.0
SALT (g)	1.09

VARIATIONS
Herbs like dill, chives, parsley and thyme are delicious in scrambled eggs, as are greens like chard, spring onions and courgettes.

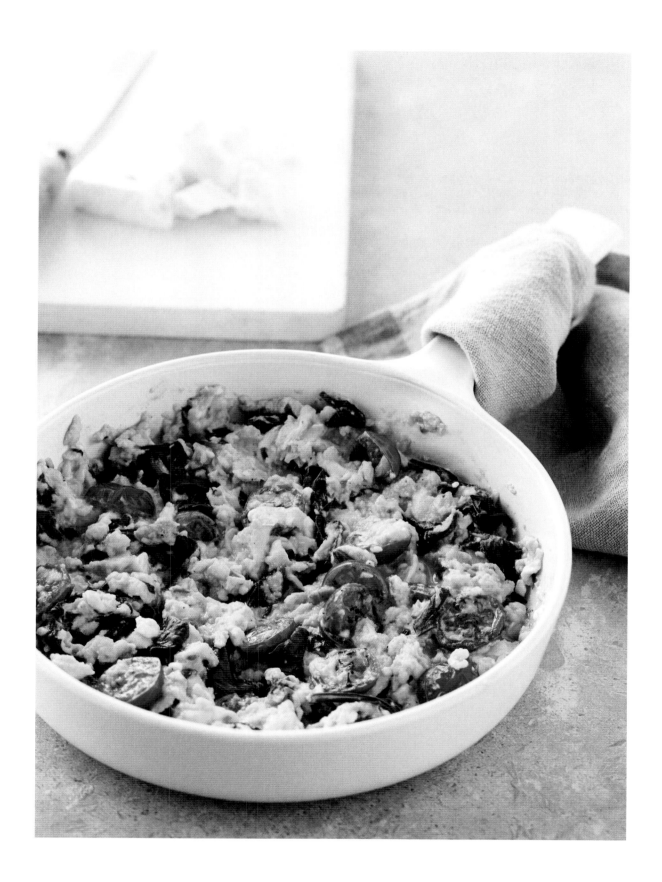

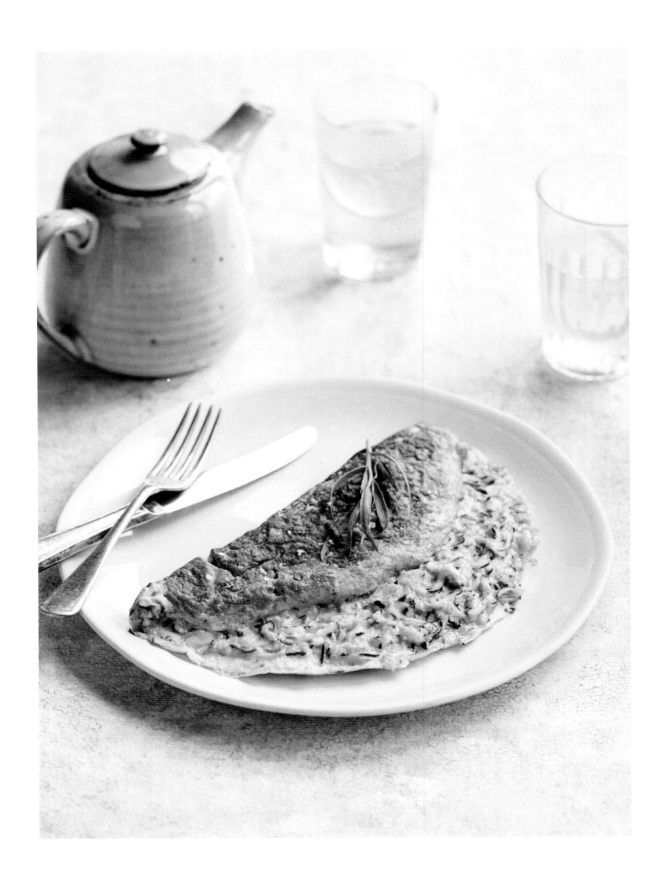

COURGETTE OMELETTE

SERVES 1

When you're trying to lose weight, eating eggs for breakfast is a really good habit to get into. Recent research has found that people who start their day with two eggs eat fewer calories over the day that follows and lose more weight than those who eat a regular carb-loaded breakfast. This omelette is ideal for one person, and packing it with courgette makes it even more filling and satisfying.

1 medium courgette, grated
Olive oil, for frying
1 tarragon sprig, leaves finely chopped
2 eggs
Sea salt and freshly ground black pepper

1. Squeeze the grated courgette to remove any excess water, then place a medium heavy-based frying pan over a medium heat and add a dash of oil. When hot, add the grated courgette and chopped tarragon and gently stir for 3–4 minutes until the courgette has softened.

2. Meanwhile, lightly beat the eggs with a fork and season with salt and pepper. Once the courgette has softened, tip out any excess liquid, then return the pan to the heat and pour in the eggs. Quickly stir and shake the pan to distribute the egg, leave to cook for 3–4 minutes until the egg is almost set, then remove from the heat.

3. With a heatproof spatula or a palette knife, loosen the sides of the omelette from the pan. Tip the pan slightly and coax the loosened edge down towards the bottom of the pan, folding the omelette in half. Next, slide or turn it out on to a serving plate and serve immediately.

PER SERVING	
KCAL	234
FAT (g)	16.0
SATURATES (g)	4.0
CARBS (g)	3.0
SUGARS (g)	2.0
FIBRE (g)	2.0
PROTEIN (g)	20.0
SALT (g)	0.52

FOR ACTIVE DAYS
If you want a great protein boost after a long workout, run or race, make this omelette with three eggs instead of two, or add an extra egg white.

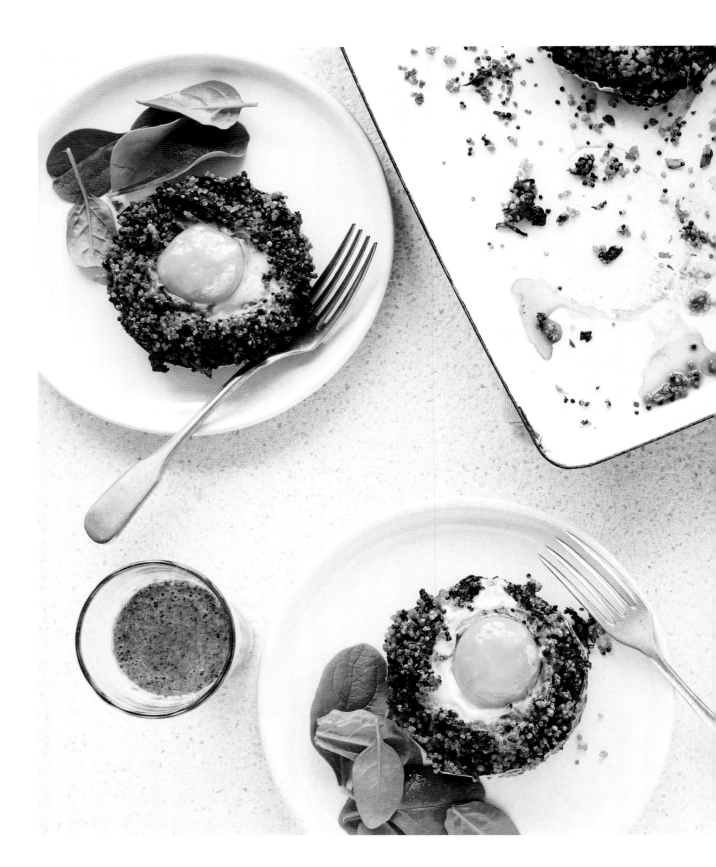

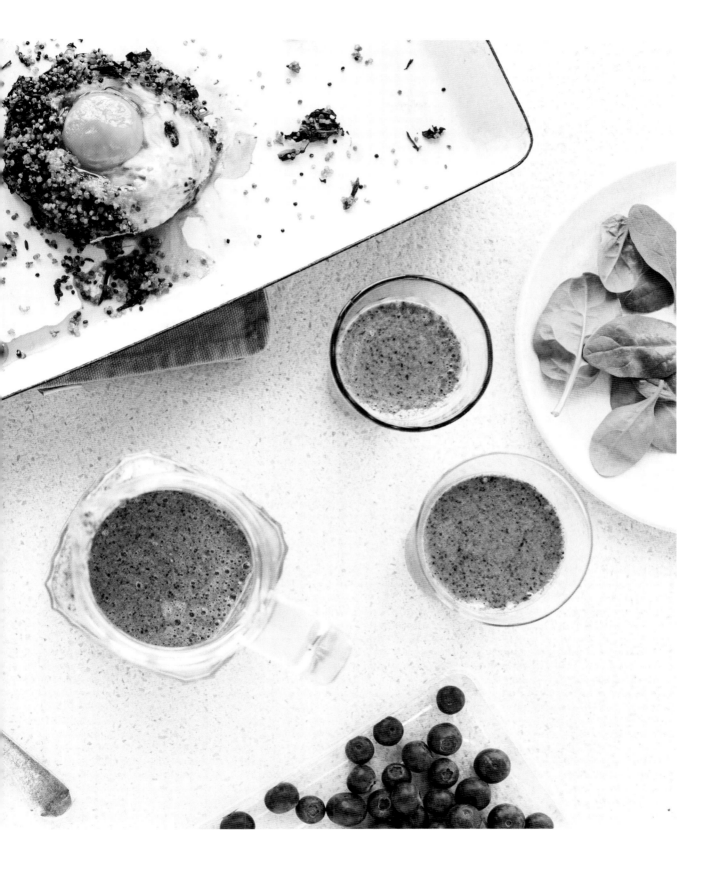

QUINOA-STUFFED MUSHROOMS WITH BAKED EGGS

SERVES 4

Eggs are packed with protein and good-for-you fats, as well as B vitamins, vitamin D, zinc and iron, and baking them inside whole mushrooms like this is really simple and very tasty. All the juices get absorbed by the mushrooms and quinoa and the slow-cooked eggs stay soft and runny. These are brilliant for a vegetarian breakfast or weekend brunch, or even lunch. It's one of those recipes that take a bit of time but not much effort, so you can get on with mixing up a virgin Mary to go with it.

4 large whole Portobello mushrooms, stalks removed and finely diced
Olive oil, for drizzling and frying
1 garlic clove, peeled and finely chopped
100g baby leaf spinach, finely shredded
175g cooked quinoa (from approximately 60g uncooked quinoa)
1 thyme sprig, leaves picked
4 small eggs
Sea salt and freshly ground black pepper

1. Preheat the oven to 180°C/gas 4.

2. Place the mushrooms gill side down on a baking tray, drizzle each one with a little olive oil and season with a pinch of salt and pepper. Put the tray into the preheated oven and cook for 5 minutes.

3. Meanwhile, heat a frying pan over a medium heat and add a dash of olive oil. When hot, sauté the chopped mushroom stalks with a pinch of salt for 3–4 minutes, until soft. Add the garlic and spinach to the pan and sauté for 3–4 minutes, until wilted.

4. Stir in the cooked quinoa and the thyme leaves.

5. Remove the mushrooms from the oven and turn them over so that the cups are facing upwards. Flatten the gills down with the back of a spoon and fill with the quinoa and spinach mixture.

6. Create a small dip in the middle of each mushroom and carefully break an egg into each dip.

7. Put the tray back into the oven for 10–12 minutes, until the whites are cooked through and the yolks are still runny. Serve immediately.

PER SERVING	
KCAL	176
FAT (g)	9.0
SATURATES (g)	2.0
CARBS (g)	10.0
SUGARS (g)	2.0
FIBRE (g)	3.0
PROTEIN (g)	12.0
SALT (g)	0.26

TOFU AND KALE SCRAMBLE

SERVES 4

I must admit that chefs don't always have good things to say about tofu! It always seems a bit spongy and tasteless, but spending time in LA where healthy eating is almost a religion, I have learnt that there are ways of making it really tasty. And the nutritional benefits are worth overcoming any mental blocks for – it's full of protein, iron and other nutrients and very low fat at the same time.

1 tbsp olive oil
1 small red onion, peeled and finely sliced
200g chestnut mushrooms, sliced
1 garlic clove, peeled and finely chopped
150g kale, roughly chopped
250g firm tofu, drained, patted dry and crumbled
½–1 tbsp soy sauce
Pinch of turmeric
Dried chilli flakes, to taste (optional)
Sea salt and freshly ground black pepper

1. Place a large frying pan over a medium heat and add the olive oil. Once hot, sweat the onion with a pinch of salt for 5–6 minutes, until soft.

2. Add the mushrooms and cook for 3–4 minutes, until soft and beginning to lightly colour. Add the garlic, stir and cook for 1 more minute.

3. Stir in the chopped kale and add 2 tablespoons of water. Cover and leave for 5 minutes, until the kale has completely wilted. Remove the lid and stir.

4. Mix in the crumbled tofu and add the soy sauce, turmeric and a pinch of chilli flakes, if using. Season with salt and pepper, then stir-fry over a medium-high heat for 2–3 minutes, until warmed through completely. Taste and add a little extra soy sauce and seasoning if needed.

5. Remove the pan from the heat and serve immediately.

FOR ACTIVE DAYS
Serve on wholemeal or rye toast before exercise, or with Sweet Potato Chips (see page 241) the night before a big day.

PER SERVING	
KCAL	159
FAT (g)	9.0
SATURATES (g)	1.0
CARBS (g)	6.0
SUGARS (g)	1.0
FIBRE (g)	2.0
PROTEIN (g)	13.0
SALT (g)	0.32

LIGHT LUNCHES TO KEEP YOU ON TRACK

CHICKEN AND QUINOA SATAY RICE PAPER ROLLS

SERVES 4 (MAKES 16 ROLLS)

Filled with lean chicken, quinoa, raw vegetables and a punchy satay sauce, these are a great take on Vietnamese summer rolls and are a firm favourite in the Ramsay house. This combination is packed with protein, making these rolls ideal for the middle of the day because protein helps stave off mid-afternoon sugar cravings. You can swap the chicken for tuna, prawns or tofu, and vary the vegetables depending on what you have. The rolls will keep for a couple of days in the fridge, so they are ideal to make ahead to take to work or on a picnic.

75g quinoa, rinsed
1 skinless chicken breast
16 x 22cm round rice paper sheets
4 mint sprigs, leaves only
1 red pepper, deseeded and finely sliced
1 courgette, julienned
1 ripe avocado, peeled, stoned and sliced
2 spring onions, finely shredded
Juice of 1 lime

FOR THE SATAY SAUCE

2 tbsp sugar-free peanut butter, smooth or crunchy
1½ tsp soy sauce
1 tsp agave syrup or runny honey
Pinch of dried chilli flakes, to taste
1 tsp rice vinegar
½ tsp freshly grated ginger

CONTINUED OVERLEAF

PER SERVING	
KCAL	387
FAT (g)	13.0
SATURATES (g)	3.0
CARBS (g)	49.0
SUGARS (g)	6.0
FIBRE (g)	5.0
PROTEIN (g)	17.0
SALT (g)	1.52

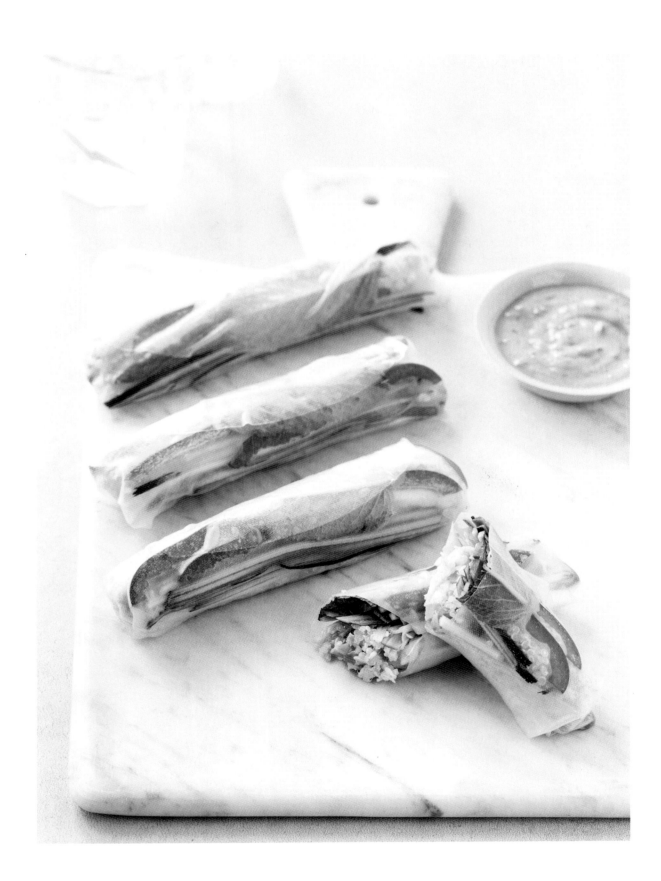

CONTINUED FROM PAGE 128

1. Cook the quinoa in a small pan of boiling water according to the packet instructions. Drain and leave to one side to cool.

2. Poach the chicken breast in a medium saucepan of hot simmering water for 15 minutes. Once cooked, remove the breast from the water and leave to cool.

3. In the meantime, make the satay sauce; mix together all the ingredients in a small bowl with a fork and let down with a teaspoon at a time of warm water until you reach a dipping consistency (approximately 5–7 teaspoons of water). The mixture will look like it's splitting at first, but if you slowly mix it with a fork it will come together and thicken as you mix. Taste and adjust the flavours as necessary.

4. Once the chicken has cooled, tear the breast into thin strips.

5. To make the rolls, place a rice paper sheet in a bowl of warm water for about 10–15 seconds, or until soft and pliable. Place it on a chopping board, then put a mint leaf in the centre and top with a couple of pieces of red pepper, courgette, avocado and spring onion. Add a tablespoon of the cooked quinoa and a couple of strips of chicken, then drizzle a little lime juice over the top.

6. Fold the sides of the rice paper over the filling, then, rolling from the bottom, using your fingers to keep the filling tightly encased, roll up tightly into a spring roll shape and repeat with the remaining ingredients.

7. Serve the rolls with the dipping sauce on the side.

GOOD TO KNOW
Rice paper is low in fat and calories and therefore a better lunch option than bread when you are trying to lose weight. Raw vegetables add colour and crunch as well as lots of nutrients that are lost when they are cooked.

LENTIL, CARROT AND CORIANDER SOUP

SERVES 4

When you are trying to lose weight, soup is like a secret weapon . . . it's low in calories but more filling than eating the same ingredients 'dry', due to the water content. This warming lentil soup is comforting and wholesome and will help keep you on track, as it keeps hunger at bay for much longer than salad. It's important to 'cook out' the garam masala to get the best flavour, so don't add the grated carrots until the aromas from the spices are released and the room is full of wonderful smells.

2 tbsp olive oil
1 red onion, peeled and diced
1 garlic clove, peeled and roughly chopped
3cm piece of fresh root ginger, peeled and roughly chopped
Bunch of coriander, leaves picked and stalks reserved
1 tbsp garam masala
500g carrots, grated
175g red lentils
1.5 litre vegetable stock
1 red chilli, deseeded and finely sliced

TO SERVE
4 tbsp low-fat yoghurt
1 lemon, quartered

1. Place a large saucepan over a medium–high heat and add the oil. When hot, add the onion, garlic and ginger.

2. Finely chop the coriander stalks and add them to the pan. Sweat the ingredients for 5 minutes.

3. Sprinkle in the garam masala and cook for 30 seconds, stirring almost constantly, then add the grated carrots and stir well.

4. Add the lentils and stock and bring to the boil. Reduce the heat and simmer for about 35 minutes, or until all the ingredients are completely soft.

5. Roughly chop the coriander leaves, then serve the soup in warmed bowls, topped with a sprinkle of coriander and chilli and a good dollop of yoghurt, with a wedge of lemon on the side.

PER SERVING	
KCAL	305
FAT (g)	8.0
SATURATES (g)	1.0
CARBS (g)	40.0
SUGARS (g)	15.0
FIBRE (g)	11.0
PROTEIN (g)	13.0
SALT (g)	1.08

HARISSA HOUMOUS
WITH CARROT ON RYE

SERVES 4

Eating more beans and pulses is really helpful when you are trying to lose weight, because they give you lots of filling fibre and protein without too many calories. Strong flavours help too, and I often reach for chilli in some form or another, not least because it is said to raise your metabolism and help burn fat. Harissa is a hot, aromatic chilli paste from North Africa that livens up marinades, rubs, dressings and pasta sauces. You could also blend some leafy vegetables like spinach or chard through the houmous for added greens.

1 x 400g tin white beans such as cannellini
  or butter beans, drained and rinsed
1 garlic clove, peeled and roughly chopped
Juice of ½ lemon
½ tsp ground cumin
½ tbsp harissa paste
1 tbsp tahini
1 tbsp extra virgin olive oil
Sea salt and freshly ground black pepper

TO SERVE
8 slices of rye or pumpernickel bread
3 carrots, grated
Chopped chives

1. Put the drained beans, garlic, lemon juice, cumin, harissa paste, tahini and a little salt and pepper into a small food processor and blend until almost smooth but still with a little texture.

2. With the motor running, slowly pour in the olive oil. Taste and adjust the seasoning as needed. Add more harissa paste if you like it a little hotter.

3. Spread the houmous on the 8 slices of bread. Add the grated carrot to 4 of the slices, sprinkle with chives, and put the other 4 slices on top. Slice the sandwiches in half and eat immediately, or wrap in cling film to take with you.

PER SERVING	
KCAL	260
FAT (g)	7.0
SATURATES (g)	1.0
CARBS (g)	34.0
SUGARS (g)	6.0
FIBRE (g)	10.0
PROTEIN (g)	10.0
SALT (g)	0.82

GOOD TO KNOW
As many of the nutrients in carrots are found in the skin or just under it, it makes sense not to peel them, but make sure you give them a really good scrub before serving them raw.

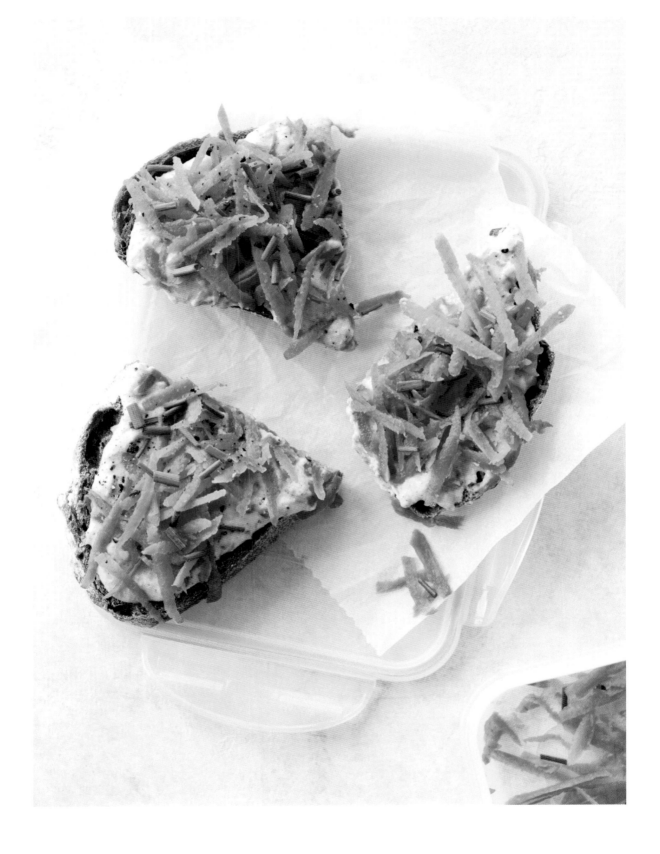

EGG 'MAYONNAISE' AND SPINACH SANDWICH

SERVES 4

Lose the real mayonnaise and you turn this sandwich into a much lighter choice than a shop-bought egg sarnie. You can still add all the traditional mayo flavourings such as a squeeze of lemon juice or vinegar and a little dash of mustard but the base is much healthier than the oil and egg yolks of a standard mayonnaise. This is delicious with the addition of finely diced gherkins, too.

6 eggs
4 tbsp natural or Greek yoghurt
1½ tsp cider vinegar
1 tsp Dijon mustard
Squeeze of lemon juice
3 dill sprigs, finely chopped
2 celery sticks, finely diced
8 slices of wholemeal bread
4 handfuls of baby spinach leaves, washed
Sea salt and freshly ground black pepper

1. Bring a large saucepan of water to the boil and, once boiling, gently add the eggs. Boil for 10 minutes then remove them from the water and put them into a bowl of cold water with ice until cool.

2. Meanwhile, put the yoghurt, vinegar, mustard, lemon juice and chopped dill into a large mixing bowl. Season with salt and pepper and stir everything together until well combined.

3. Once the eggs are cool, peel and dice them or mash with a fork then add to the yoghurt mix with the celery. Mix everything together. Taste and adjust the seasoning as necessary.

4. Divide the egg mixture between the 8 slices of bread and top 4 of the slices with a handful of spinach. Place the remaining slices on top and cut the sandwiches in half to serve or wrap in cling film and store in the fridge for later.

PER SERVING	
KCAL	399
FAT (g)	15.0
SATURATES (g)	6.0
CARBS (g)	26.0
SUGARS (g)	4.0
FIBRE (g)	5.0
PROTEIN (g)	22.0
SALT (g)	1.2

BROWN RICE SUSHI HAND ROLLS

SERVES 4 (MAKES 8 HAND ROLLS)

I absolutely love Japanese food, and it is always a great choice when you are trying to lose weight because the ingredients and cooking methods are naturally low in fat and nutrient-rich. What's more, the sauces and seasonings are strong and satisfying – diet food should never be boring. Hand rolls look impressive but are actually quite easy to put together. I've used smoked salmon in this recipe because it's easy to get hold of, but if you have access to a brilliant fishmonger and really fresh, sushi-grade fish, then go down the more traditional route and make these with raw salmon or tuna.

115g brown sushi rice or short-grain brown rice
1½ tbsp mirin
1½ tbsp rice vinegar
4 sheets of sushi nori seaweed
150g sliced smoked salmon, torn into
  bite-sized pieces
1 ripe avocado, peeled, stoned and cubed
½ cucumber, cut into batons
2 tbsp sesame seeds, black or white
100g sushi ginger
Sea salt
Soy sauce, to serve

CONTINUED OVERLEAF

GOOD TO KNOW
Seaweed, like nori, is very nutrient-dense and is especially valued for its high mineral content, including iodine, which is essential for a healthy metabolism.

PER SERVING	
KCAL	299
FAT (g)	14.0
SATURATES (g)	3.0
CARBS (g)	27.0
SUGARS (g)	3.0
FIBRE (g)	4.0
PROTEIN (g)	14.0
SALT (g)	1.40

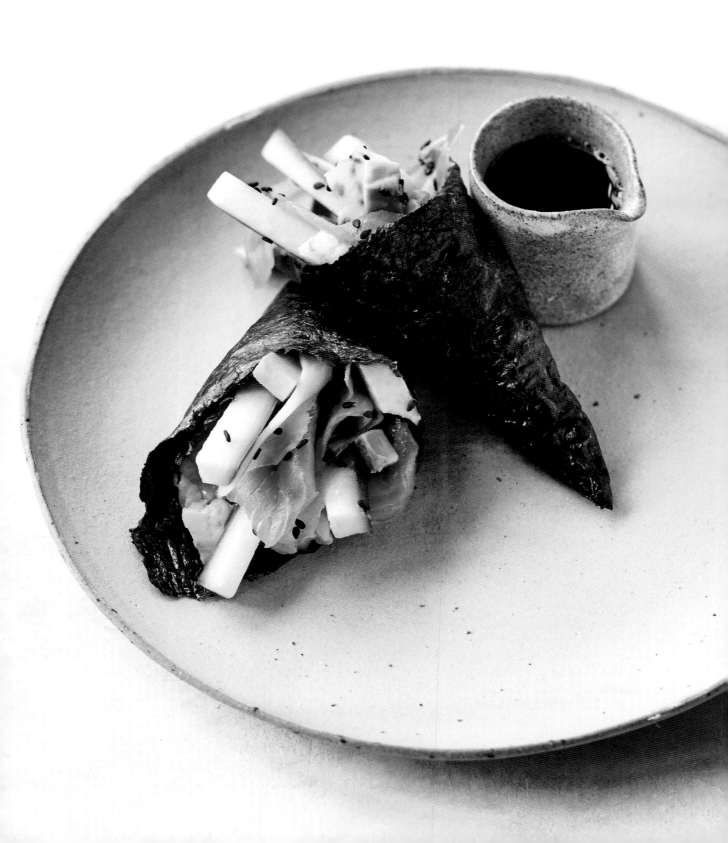

CONTINUED FROM PAGE 135

1. Rinse the rice really well in a sieve under cold running water until the water runs clear.

2. Put the rice into a medium saucepan with a tight-fitting lid and pour over 250ml of water. Bring the pan to a simmer, then reduce the heat to low. Put the lid on and leave the pan for 30 minutes over a low heat without removing the lid, until all the water has been absorbed and the rice is tender. Remove the pan from the heat and leave to stand for 10 minutes with the lid still on.

3. After 10 minutes, spread the rice on a clean tray and sprinkle over the mirin, rice vinegar and a couple of pinches of salt. Mix the rice together to make sure everything is coated, and spread out to cool at room temperature.

4. Once the rice has cooled and you are ready to assemble the hand rolls, cut the nori sheets in half, then fill a small bowl with warm water. Place one piece of seaweed on a board with the long side facing towards you. Add 1 tablespoon of rice to the middle of the right-hand half of the sheet. Wet your hands and press the rice down gently to flatten it. Place a couple of pieces of salmon on the rice and top with avocado, cucumber, a sprinkling of sesame seeds and a couple of pieces of sushi ginger. The top right corner will be the open end, so place the cucumber batons with one end at that corner to make it easier to roll.

5. Take the bottom right corner of the nori sheet and fold it over so that it covers the filling and is now at the top left corner of the right half of the nori sheet. You should have an opening where the top right corner was. Now, with your fingers securing the nori sheet covering the filling, roll tightly towards the empty left-hand side of the sheet to create a tight cone shape. The bottom left corner of the right-hand half of the sheet will be the point at which you pivot the cone from. Wet the edge of the nori sheet with your fingers and stick it to the cone, securing the nori tightly. Repeat with the remaining sheets and filling.

6. Serve the hand rolls with soy sauce on the side.

VARIATION
If you can't get hold of brown sushi rice or brown short-grain rice, then replace with white sushi rice. However, this rice will not be as sticky, so make sure to wrap your hand rolls tightly to avoid the contents spilling out.

CHICKEN AND KALE CAESAR SALAD

SERVES 4

Massaging kale sounds like a crazy thing to do but it actually tenderizes the leaves, making them soft enough to eat without having to cook them. You can also dress this salad up to two days in advance, which will tenderize the leaves further. If you miss the croutons in a classic Caesar salad, try sprinkling Crunchy Chickpeas over the top instead (see page 99).

350g kale, stalks removed and leaves shredded
Olive oil
2 skinless chicken breasts, butterflied
1 head of red chicory, leaves separated
Sea salt and freshly ground black pepper

FOR THE DRESSING
1 garlic clove, peeled and roughly chopped
4 anchovy fillets, drained and roughly chopped
½ tsp Dijon mustard
2 tbsp grated Parmesan cheese, plus extra
   for serving (optional)
Juice of ¼–½ lemon, to taste
1 tbsp extra virgin olive oil
150g natural yoghurt

1. Put the shredded kale into a large mixing bowl, season with salt and pepper and drizzle with the olive oil. Rub the oil and seasoning into the kale leaves for a few minutes to help tenderize the leaves, then leave for 30 minutes while you prepare the rest of the salad.

2. Heat a griddle pan over a medium–high heat. Rub the butterflied chicken breasts with a little olive oil and season with salt and pepper. Place on the griddle pan for 3–4 minutes on each side, or until just cooked through. Remove the chicken and leave to rest.

3. Meanwhile, make the dressing; put all the ingredients into a blender and blitz until smooth. Taste and adjust the seasoning, adding a little more lemon juice, if needed.

4. Once the chicken has cooled and the kale is tenderized, toss the kale and chicory with the dressing, mixing really well to coat the leaves. Slice the chicken, place it on top, then grate over a little Parmesan, if using.

PER SERVING	
KCAL	241
FAT (g)	12.0
SATURATES (g)	3.0
CARBS (g)	5.0
SUGARS (g)	4.0
FIBRE (g)	4.0
PROTEIN (g)	28.0
SALT (g)	0.92

HOW TO SOFTEN KALE
If you don't have time to massage and marinate the kale leaves, you can also blanch them very briefly in boiling water, then refresh them in iced water and dry thoroughly.

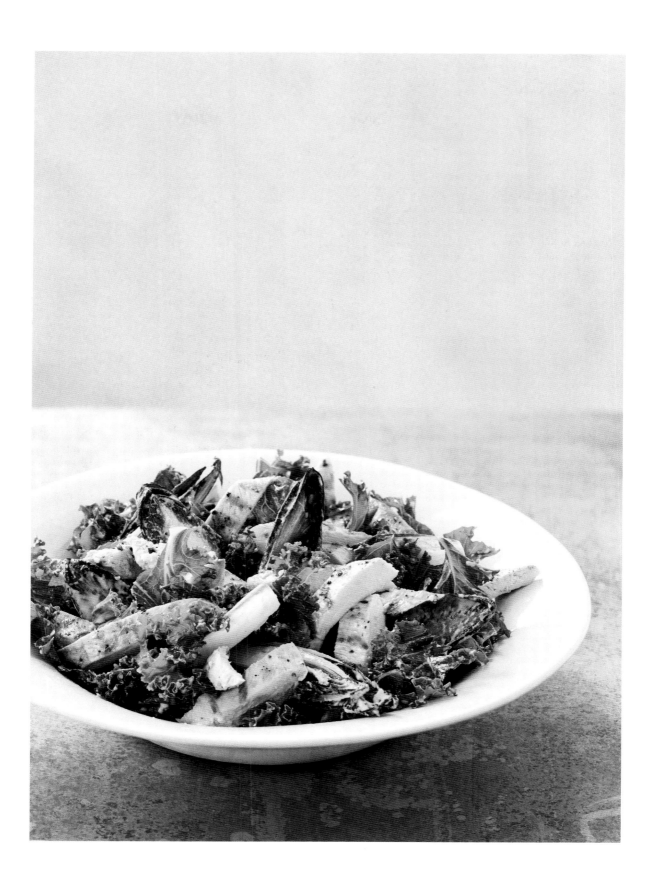

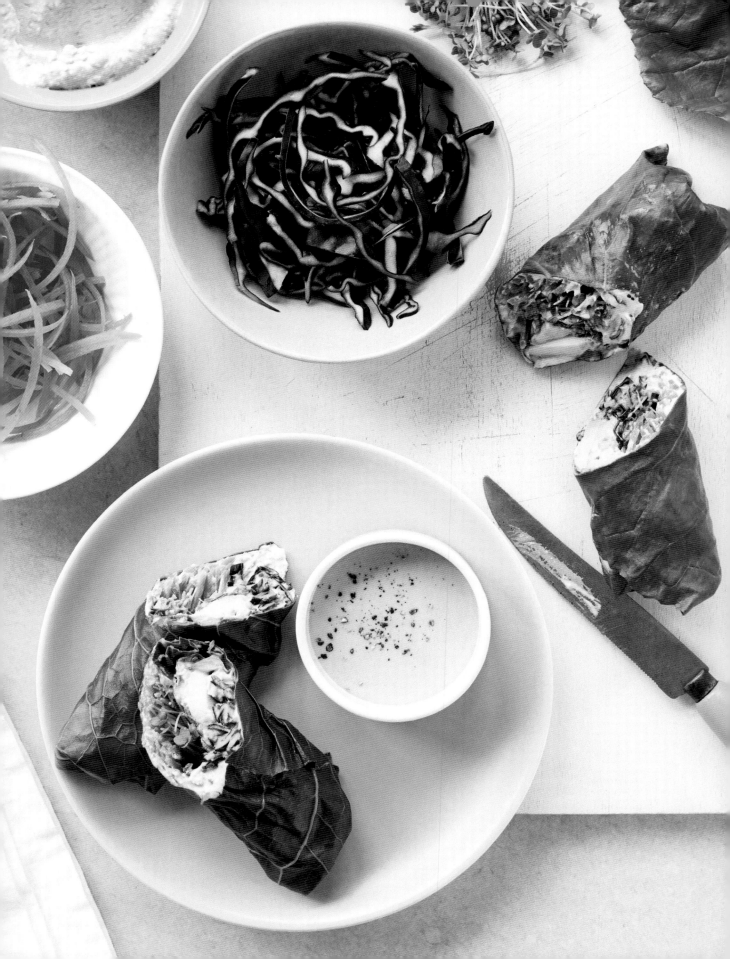

SPRING GREEN WRAPS

SERVES 4 (MAKES 8 WRAPS)

Using cabbage leaves to make wraps is an ingenious way of upping your vegetable intake. They have a lovely crunchy texture and work surprisingly well in place of a tortilla or rice paper wrap. In the States these are often made with the leaves of collard greens, but in the UK the closest vegetable we have to this is spring greens. You could also use hispi, pointed or Savoy cabbage leaves, or swap the leaves for wholemeal or seeded tortilla wraps if you are trying to get in some carbs before exercise.

8 large, outer spring green leaves
200g houmous
2 carrots, grated
¼ small red cabbage, very finely shredded
1 ripe avocado, peeled, stoned and sliced
1 punnet of salad cress, snipped

FOR THE DRESSING/DIPPING SAUCE
4 tbsp tahini
1 tbsp soy sauce
2 tsp maple syrup or runny honey
Juice of 1 lime
Sea salt and freshly ground black pepper

1. To make the dressing/dipping sauce, put all the ingredients into a bowl with a pinch of salt and pepper. Mix well until completely combined, then add warm water 1 teaspoon at a time, mixing after each addition until you reach a drizzling/dipping consistency.

2. Heat a medium frying pan three-quarters full of hot water and bring to a simmer. Cut the woody stem from the very bottom of each spring green leaf, leaving as much of the leaf as possible intact. Dip each leaf, one at a time, into the hot water for 10 seconds or until wilted and bright green in colour. Remove and leave to one side.

3. Spread the leaves out on a board. Divide the houmous between the leaves and spread it out.

4. Arrange a little grated carrot, shredded red cabbage, sliced avocado and cress in the middle of each leaf. Drizzle each pile of vegetables with a little dressing, then fold the sides of the leaves inwards over the filling and roll up from the bottom, enclosing the mixture completely.

5. Place the wraps, edge side down, on a board and slice them diagonally through the middle, then serve with the dipping sauce in a bowl on the side.

HOW TO SOFTEN CABBAGE LEAVES
If you don't have time to blanch the cabbage leaves, you can put them in the microwave for 10–12 seconds to soften them.

PER SERVING	
KCAL	331
FAT (g)	23.0
SATURATES (g)	4.0
CARBS (g)	17.0
SUGARS (g)	8.0
FIBRE (g)	9.0
PROTEIN (g)	9.0
SALT (g)	0.90

LEAN SUPPERS AND SIDES

MEXICAN PRAWN COCKTAIL

SERVES 4

Unlike a traditional British prawn cocktail, which
is smothered in mayonnaise, the Mexican version
is made with a tangy tomato-based sauce spiked
with lime and chilli. It's quite different and much
more refreshing – my family are total converts.
Serve as a starter with Pitta Crisps (see page 266)
for added crunch, or unsalted tortillas if you aren't
trying to be lean.

1½ tbsp tomato ketchup
Juice of ½ orange
1 tsp Worcestershire sauce
Juice of 1 lime
½ small bunch of coriander, leaves and
   stalks roughly chopped
4 medium tomatoes, diced
1 small white onion, peeled and finely diced
1 cucumber, finely diced
400g cooked king prawns, peeled and
   deveined if necessary
1 ripe avocado, peeled, stoned and diced
Sea salt and freshly ground black pepper

TO SERVE
1 lime, quartered
Mexican hot sauce such as Cholula (optional)

1. In a large mixing bowl, combine the tomato
ketchup, orange juice, Worcestershire sauce and lime
juice and mix until thoroughly combined. Add the
coriander leaves and stalks, tomatoes, onion and
cucumber and mix well. Season with a little salt
and pepper.

2. Stir in the prawns and coat with the sauce.
Taste and adjust the seasoning as necessary.

3. Serve the prawn cocktail in cocktail glasses or small
bowls, with the avocado sprinkled over the top and
a lime wedge on the side. This is delicious with a few
drops of Mexican hot sauce on top.

PER SERVING	
KCAL	185
FAT (g)	8.0
SATURATES (g)	2.0
CARBS (g)	8.0
SUGARS (g)	7.0
FIBRE (g)	4.0
PROTEIN (g)	19.0
SALT (g)	1.79

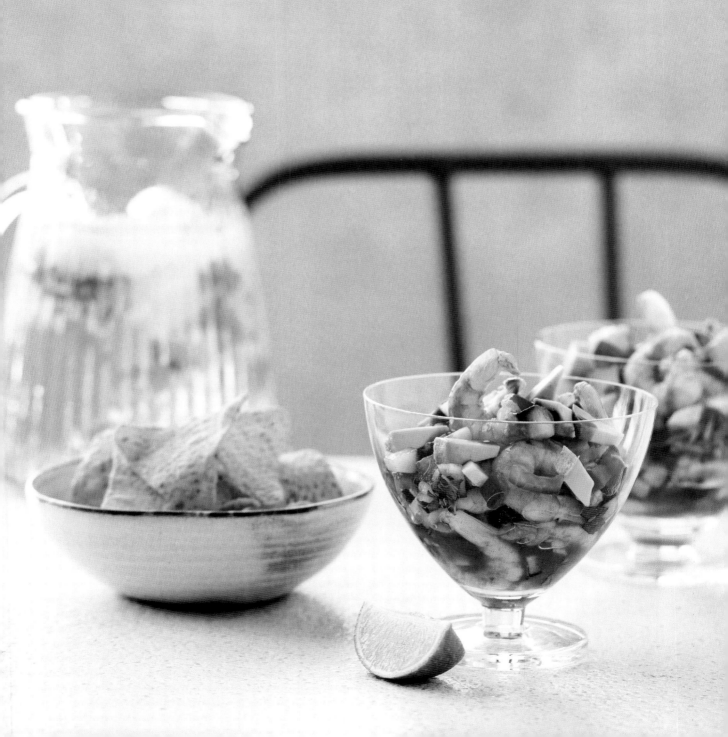

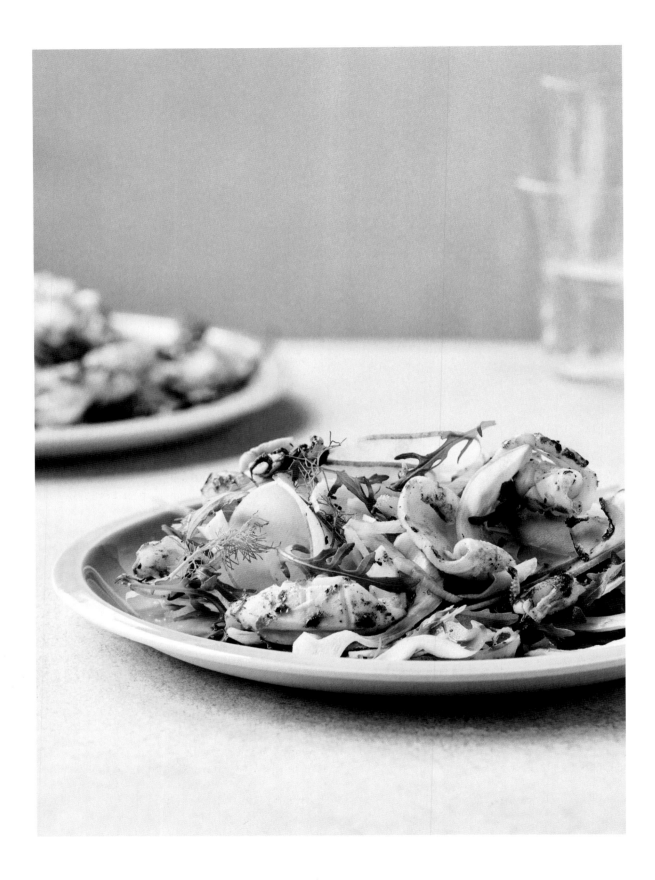

GRILLED SQUID, FENNEL AND APPLE SALAD
SERVES 4

Squid should either be cooked very fast or very slow – anything in between and you will feel like you're tucking into a plate of rubber bands. So when I say cook for 1 minute on each side, that's exactly what I mean . . . this should be just long enough for the flesh to turn opaque but still stay tender. When you're not trying hard to be lean, a little fried chorizo added to this salad is absolutely delicious.

4 medium squid (approx. 400g), prepared and cleaned
Olive oil, for drizzling
1 tsp smoked paprika
1 large fennel bulb
1 large sharp eating apple such as Granny Smith, cored
Juice of 1 lemon
150g rocket leaves
2 mint sprigs, leaves roughly torn
Sherry vinegar
Sea salt and freshly ground black pepper

1. Slice the squid tubes open and lightly score one side in a diamond pattern before slicing each tube into 6 pieces. Cut any large tentacles into smaller bite-sized pieces and place everything in a medium mixing bowl. Drizzle with olive oil, and sprinkle over the smoked paprika and a pinch of salt and pepper. Toss to make sure everything is coated with smoked paprika and put to one side.

2. Meanwhile, finely slice the fennel and apple, ideally on a mandolin or with a very sharp knife. Put the slices into a bowl of cold water with the lemon juice to prevent them turning brown.

3. Heat a griddle pan over a high heat. Once hot, add the squid, in batches if necessary, and cook for about 1 minute on each side until lightly charred and just cooked through.

4. Drain the fennel and apple and pat dry with a clean tea towel or kitchen paper. Put the slices on to a serving plate and mix in the rocket and the torn mint leaves. Drizzle with a little olive oil, sherry vinegar and a pinch of salt and pepper, then place the hot squid on top and sprinkle with a few extra dots of sherry vinegar. Serve immediately.

HOW TO BARBECUE SQUID
You could also grill the squid on the barbecue for a more charred, smoky flavour. Cut the flesh into slightly bigger pieces so that they don't fall through the gaps in the grill, and cook for 1 minute on each side.

PER SERVING	
KCAL	180
FAT (g)	8.0
SATURATES (g)	1.0
CARBS (g)	6.0
SUGARS (g)	6.0
FIBRE (g)	5.0
PROTEIN (g)	18.0
SALT (g)	0.34

SALMON CEVICHE WITH GRAPEFRUIT, AVOCADO AND MINT

SERVES 4

This salmon ceviche is a simple but smart dish to serve when you are watching your weight. It is low in calories but the combination of flavours is bold and satisfying, and because the fish isn't exposed to heat, it retains all of the valuable omega-3 fats which might otherwise be damaged during cooking. The bitter grapefruit juice goes brilliantly with the salmon, but you could swap it for any other meaty white fish too – just make sure that whatever fish you choose, it's as fresh as possible.

1 pink or red grapefruit
400g salmon fillet, skin and pin-bones removed, finely sliced
1 small banana shallot, peeled and finely diced
100g radishes, trimmed and finely sliced
1 ripe avocado, peeled, stoned and diced
5 mint sprigs, leaves roughly torn
Sea salt

1. Cut the grapefruit in half horizontally, then juice one of the halves. Remove the segments from the second half – do this over a bowl to collect any juices.

2. Put the sliced salmon, grapefruit juice and segments, diced shallot and radishes into a large mixing bowl and season with couple of pinches of salt. Toss well to mix and leave to stand for 10 minutes or up to 30 minutes (see tip on page 76).

3. When ready to serve, transfer the ceviche to a serving plate or shallow bowl. Fold in the avocado and sprinkle over the torn mint leaves. Taste and adjust the seasoning as necessary, and serve immediately.

PER SERVING	
KCAL	270
FAT (g)	17.0
SATURATES (g)	4.0
CARBS (g)	4.0
SUGARS (g)	3.0
FIBRE (g)	3.0
PROTEIN (g)	23.0
SALT (g)	0.14

FOR ACTIVE DAYS
If you are not counting calories, serve the ceviche with Melba toast, rye or pumpernickel bread, or the Pitta Crisps on page 266.

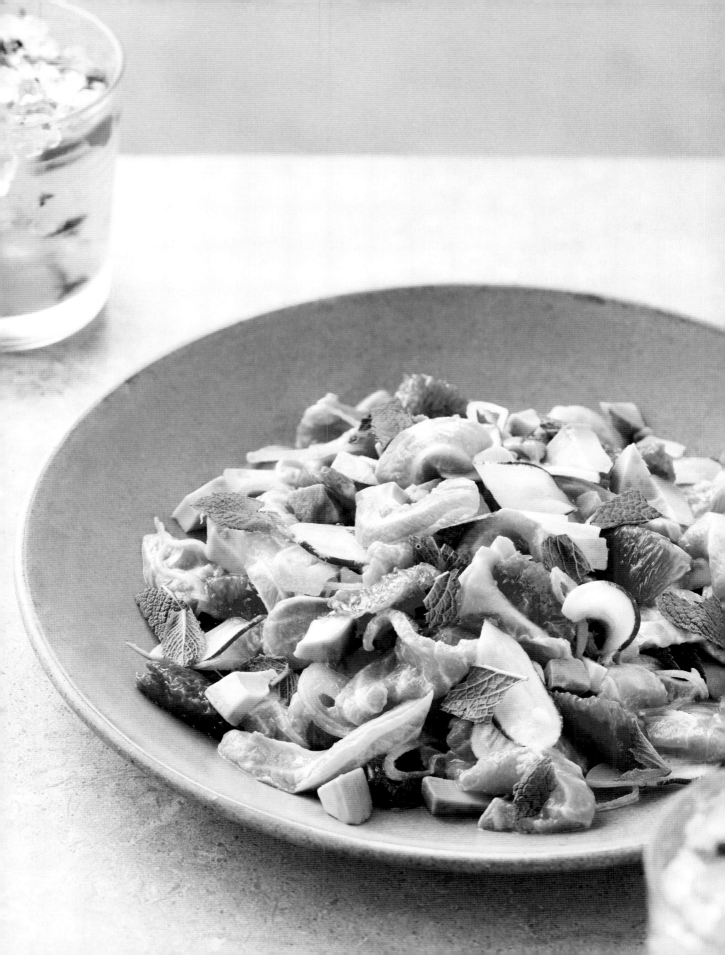

EDAMAME, BROAD BEAN AND PEA SOUP

SERVES 4

Edamame, broad beans, peas and eggs are all excellent sources of protein, making this a really filling soup that will keep you satisfied long after you have eaten it – which means no hankering for off-limits snacks. Use frozen beans and peas for this recipe so you don't have to spend time podding and shelling them before cooking.

20ml rapeseed oil
1 large onion, peeled and diced
2 celery sticks, trimmed and diced
1 medium potato, peeled and diced
2 thyme sprigs, leaves only, plus a few extra
   leaves to garnish
1 litre chicken stock
200g broad beans, podded and shelled
150g edamame beans, podded
4 eggs
100g peas
1 red chilli, deseeded and finely sliced
1½ tsp black sesame seeds

1. Place a large saucepan over a medium heat and add the rapeseed oil. When hot, add the onion, celery, potato and thyme leaves and cook for 8 minutes, stirring regularly.

2. Pour in the stock and bring to the boil. Simmer for 10 minutes, then add the broad beans and edamame beans and simmer for a further 10 minutes.

3. Meanwhile, bring a large saucepan of water up to the boil, then reduce the heat and poach the eggs for 3 minutes, until the white has set but the yolk is still runny (see below).

4. When the beans are cooked, add the peas and bring to the boil again. Blitz the ingredients with a blender.

5. Divide the soup between four warmed bowls, slide an egg in to each one, then sprinkle with red chilli, black sesame seeds and a few extra thyme leaves before serving.

PER SERVING	
KCAL	334
FAT (g)	14.0
SATURATES (g)	3.0
CARBS (g)	22.0
SUGARS (g)	7.0
FIBRE (g)	11.0
PROTEIN (g)	25.0
SALT (g)	0.89

HOW TO POACH AN EGG
Bring a large pan of water up to the boil with a little splash of vinegar, then reduce to a gentle bubble. Use a whisk to stir the water in a circle, to create a whirlpool. Crack the egg into a tea cup and slip it into the centre of the circulating water. Poach for 3 minutes, or until the egg floats to the surface, then remove from the pan and drain on kitchen paper before serving.

TAMARIND PRAWNS

SERVES 4

Tamarind has a sweet but tart flavour that goes really well with prawns and other fish. Here I am balancing the sourness with salty fish sauce and sweet agave syrup to make a distinct sweet and sour sauce that is popular across South East Asia. These prawns are lip-smackingly good as a light starter or served with brown rice and Asian greens for a main dish.

280g brown rice
3 tbsp tamarind paste or watered-down
   tamarind block (see below)
1 tbsp fish sauce, to taste
1 tbsp agave syrup, to taste
1 tbsp coconut oil, or cooking oil of your choice
1 banana shallot, peeled and finely sliced
2 garlic cloves, peeled and finely sliced
4 pak choi
400g raw king prawns, peeled and deveined
   if necessary, patted dry
½ small bunch of coriander, roughly chopped

CONTINUED OVERLEAF

HOW TO PREPARE TAMARIND
To water down a block of tamarind, soak it in a little hot water, remove the seeds, and mash it well to create a thick juice.

PER SERVING	
KCAL	434
FAT (g)	7.0
SATURATES (g)	3.0
CARBS (g)	64.0
SUGARS (g)	10.0
FIBRE (g)	5.0
PROTEIN (g)	26.0
SALT (g)	1.43

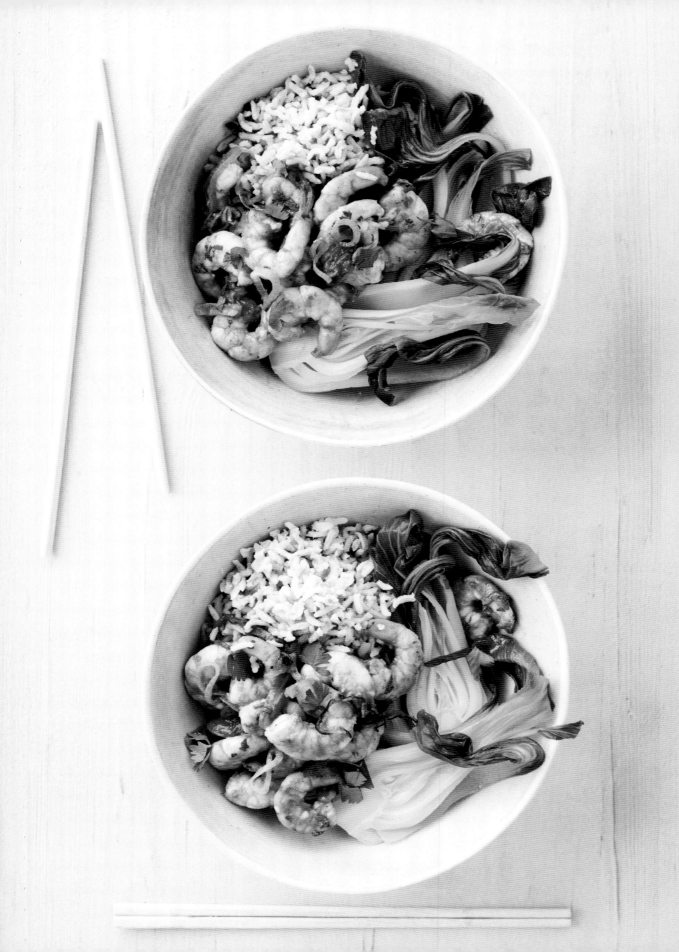

CONTINUED FROM PAGE 151

1. Rinse the rice really well in a sieve under cold running water until the water runs clear.

2. Put the rice into a medium saucepan with a tight-fitting lid and pour over 560ml of water. Bring the pan to a simmer, then reduce the heat to low. Put the lid on and leave the pan for 30 minutes over a low heat without removing the lid, until all the water has been absorbed and the rice is tender.

3. Mix the tamarind, fish sauce and agave syrup together in a separate small saucepan and place over a low heat. Stir until completely combined. Taste and adjust the sweetness and saltiness as necessary. Set aside.

4. When the rice is cooked, remove the pan from the heat and leave to stand for 10 minutes with the lid on.

5. Place a wok or a large frying pan over a high heat and add the coconut oil. Once hot, fry the shallot and garlic for 4–5 minutes, until softened and turning slightly golden on the edges.

6. Meanwhile, slice the pak choi in half lengthways and cook in a large pan of salted boiling water for 3 minutes until wilted.

7. Once the shallots are softened, add the prawns to the frying pan and stir-fry for 2 minutes, then pour over the tamarind sauce. Stir well so the prawns are well coated, then cook for a further 2–3 minutes until the prawns are cooked through and the sauce is thick enough to coat them.

8. When ready to serve, remove the lid from the rice pan and fluff up the rice with a fork.

9. Divide the rice, prawns and pak choi between four plates or bowls and garnish with the chopped coriander.

SEARED TUNA AND VEGETABLE SKEWERS WITH WASABI DIPPING SAUCE

SERVES 4

Despite being an oily fish, tuna can dry out very easily, so don't overcook these skewers – the cubes of fish should still be a little pink in the centre. You can try other vegetables here – sugar snap peas or courgette chunks would also be delicious, as would adding slivers of pickled sushi ginger between the tuna chunks. Pile up the skewers on a large plate or board and serve with the dipping sauce for everyone to help themselves, or plate them with some brown rice and the Asian Slaw (see page 156).

4 tuna steaks (approximately 140g each), cut into 2.5cm cubes
2 tbsp soy sauce
250g asparagus spears, trimmed
Flavourless oil, e.g. groundnut, for frying

FOR THE WASABI DIPPING SAUCE
1–2 tsp wasabi powder or 2 tsp wasabi paste, to taste (see below)
3 tbsp soy sauce
1 tbsp runny honey or ½ tbsp agave syrup
1 tsp sesame oil
1 tbsp rice vinegar

1. Put the tuna cubes into a bowl and pour over the soy sauce. Massage gently into the tuna and leave to marinate.

2. Blanch the asparagus in a large pan of salted boiling water for 2 minutes. Remove from the pan and refresh immediately in cold water.

3. Slice the asparagus diagonally into 3cm long pieces.

4. Mix together the ingredients for the wasabi dipping sauce, starting with 1 tsp of the wasabi powder or paste. Taste and add more if you like a stronger wasabi flavour and a little more punch.

5. Place a griddle pan or a large frying pan over a medium heat.

6. Thread the tuna cubes and asparagus alternately on to skewers (if using bamboo skewers, soak them in water for 20 minutes beforehand).

7. Drizzle a little oil on a plate and roll each skewer in the oil, then place on the hot griddle or frying pan. Cook for 2–3 minutes on each side until lightly marked but still pink in the middle (you may have to do this in batches, depending on the size of the griddle or frying pan).

8. Serve the skewers warm or at room temperature, with the dipping sauce on the side.

PER SERVING	
KCAL	241
FAT (g)	5.0
SATURATES (g)	1.0
CARBS (g)	9.0
SUGARS (g)	8.0
FIBRE (g)	1.0
PROTEIN (g)	39.0
SALT (g)	2.82

VARIATION
If you don't like wasabi, replace it with 1 teaspoon of freshly grated ginger.

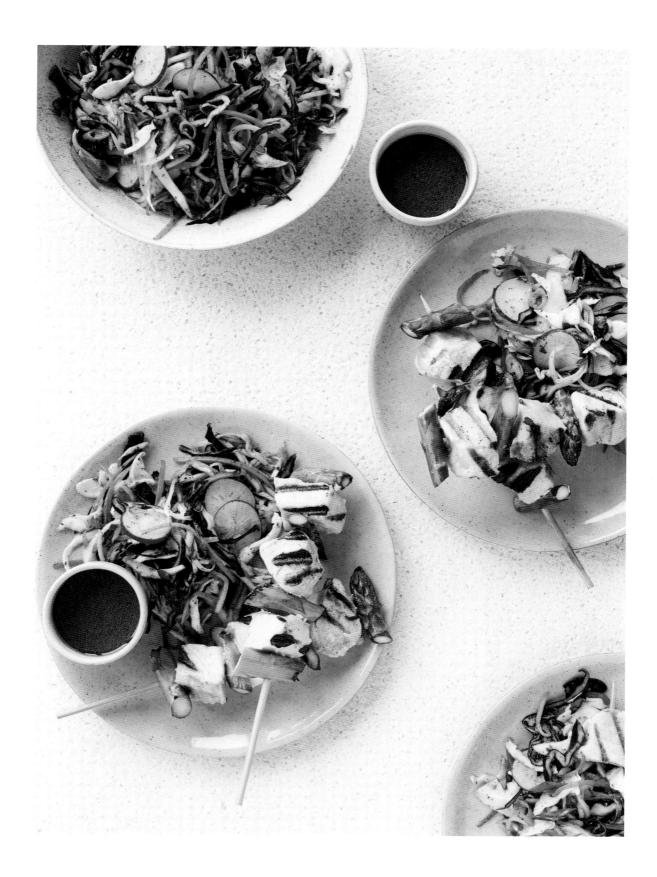

ASIAN SLAW

SERVES 4 AS A SIDE

Green mangos are unripe mangos that are still hard to the touch. They are popular in cooking across Asia and are often used in salads, curries, rice dishes, pickles and chutneys. Served raw and cut into batons, they add a tart flavour and welcome crunch to this crisp slaw. If you can't get hold of unripe mangos, use a couple of Granny Smith apples instead. Serve this with lean chicken, pork or fish to make it more filling without adding many more calories.

½ small red cabbage, core removed and leaves finely shredded
½ small white cabbage, core removed and leaves finely shredded
2 carrots, grated
100g radishes, trimmed and sliced
2 spring onions, trimmed and finely sliced
1 green mango, peeled and julienned
½–1 red chilli, deseeded and finely chopped (optional)

FOR THE DRESSING
Large bunch of coriander
1 ball of stem ginger, roughly chopped
Juice of 3 limes
½ tbsp fish sauce
½ tsp rice vinegar
2 tsp agave syrup

1. Put all the vegetables and the mango into a bowl with the chilli, if using.

2. To make the dressing, put the coriander and stem ginger into a blender and blitz until very finely chopped. Add the remaining dressing ingredients and blend until smooth. Taste and adjust the flavours as necessary.

3. Pour the dressing over the vegetables and mix really well before serving.

PER SERVING	
KCAL	105
FAT (g)	1.0
SATURATES (g)	0.1
CARBS (g)	18.0
SUGARS (g)	17.0
FIBRE (g)	7.0
PROTEIN (g)	3.0
SALT (g)	0.47

TRAY-BAKED CHICKEN WITH BUTTER BEANS, LEEKS AND SPINACH

SERVES 4–6

Cooking everything together in one pan has some great advantages – all the prep work is done up front, so you can get on with other things once it's in the oven, the flavours really come together as they cook and there is only one pan to wash up when you're finished. It makes for a great family-friendly recipe and no arguments about who's doing the dishes. Serve with roasted baby potatoes in their skins or the Sweet Potato Chips on page 241 if weight loss isn't a priority.

1 whole chicken, jointed, or 2 breasts,
  2 thighs and 2 drumsticks, skin removed
1 tbsp olive oil
1 head of garlic, cut in half horizontally
1 leek, trimmed, halved lengthways and sliced
200ml dry white wine
400ml chicken or vegetable stock
2 thyme sprigs
2 x 400g tins butter beans, drained and rinsed
250g baby spinach leaves
Sea salt and freshly ground black pepper

1. Preheat the oven to 180°C/gas 4. Season the chicken with salt and pepper.

2. Place a large roasting tray on the hob to warm up and add the oil. Once hot, brown the chicken pieces on all sides until nicely coloured. Turn the chicken skin side up.

3. Add the garlic to the tray, cut side down, then add the leeks and stir around in the oil.

4. Pour in the white wine and allow to bubble for 2 minutes, then add the stock. Use a wooden spoon to scrape up any bits stuck to the bottom.

5. Turn off the heat and add the thyme sprigs, butter beans and spinach, nestling them between the chicken pieces. Season with a pinch of salt and pepper and mix everything together, then put the tray into the preheated oven. Bake for 35–40 minutes, until the chicken is cooked through. Give the tray a stir occasionally to make sure everything is cooking evenly.

6. Remove the tray from the oven and leave to rest for 5 minutes before serving in warm shallow bowls.

TO MAKE IT LESS LEAN
Leave the skin on the chicken if you aren't watching your weight, and follow the recipe above but be careful not to pour the wine or stock over the browned skin because it won't crisp up properly in the oven.

PER SERVING	
KCAL	509
FAT (g)	16.0
SATURATES (g)	4.0
CARBS (g)	18.0
SUGARS (g)	2.0
FIBRE (g)	10.0
PROTEIN (g)	58.0
SALT (g)	0.62

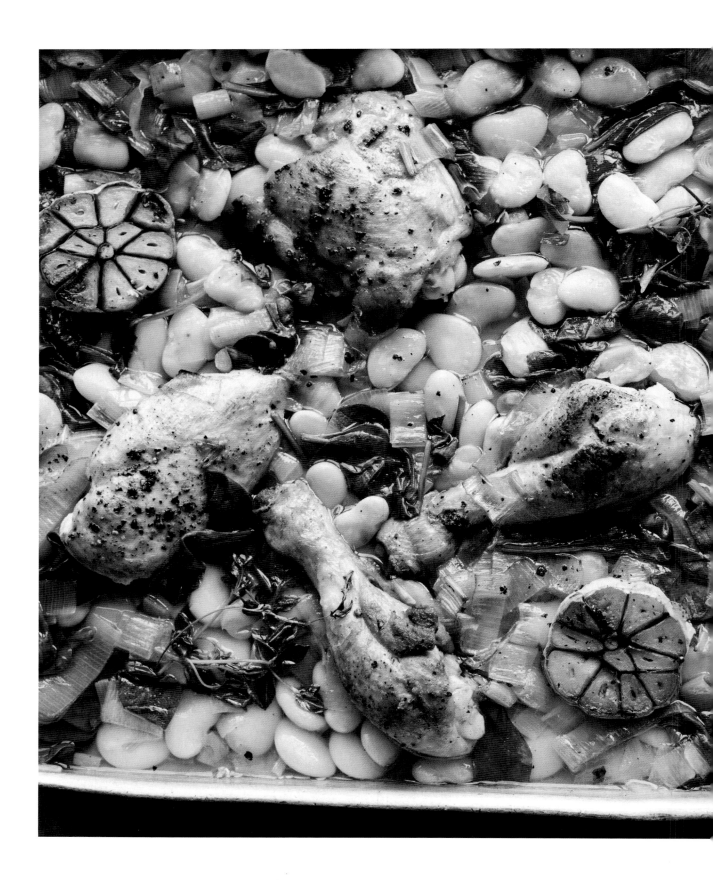

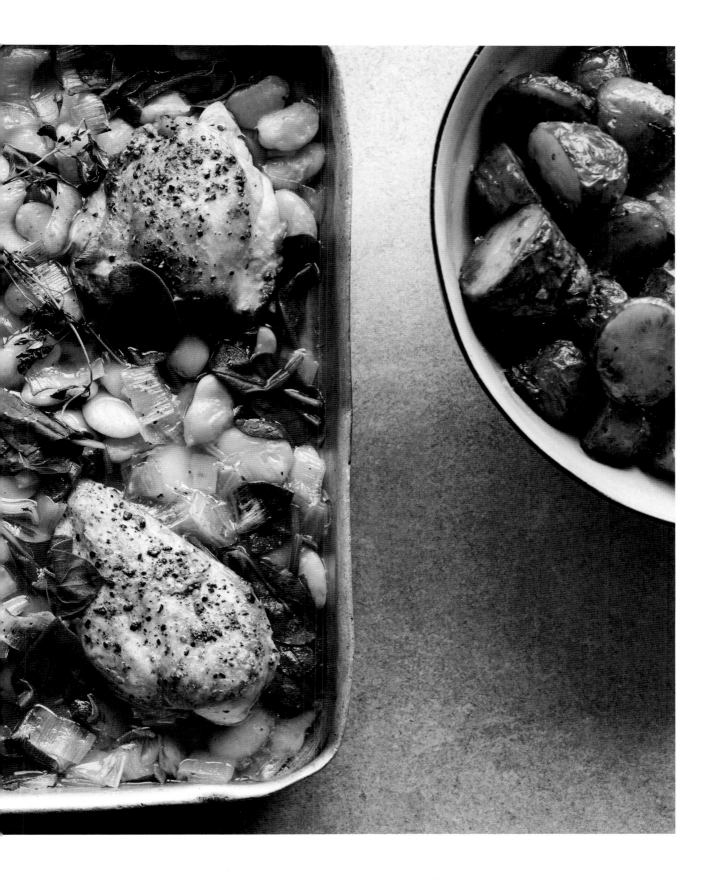

DUCK BREAST WITH BRAISED FENNEL AND ORANGE GREMOLATA

SERVES 4

Duck has a reputation of being really fatty but if you remove the skin, the breasts are actually leaner than a fillet steak and with more iron than a chicken breast. Braising fennel not only softens it, it also mellows the strong aniseed flavour of the raw vegetable while the orange gremolata adds zest and freshness. This is equally delicious served straight from the oven or at room temperature.

2 fennel bulbs
Olive oil
Juice of ½ orange (zest used below)
4 x 150g duck breasts, skin removed
    and trimmed of fat
Sea salt and freshly ground black pepper

FOR THE GREMOLATA
Zest of 1 orange (from above)
Small bunch of flat-leaf parsley, leaves
    finely chopped
1 garlic clove, peeled and very finely chopped

1. Preheat the oven to 170°C/gas 3.

2. Remove any green fronds from the fennel and reserve for serving. Slice the fennel in half lengthways, then slice each half in half again.

3. Heat a large casserole dish over a medium heat. Add a dash of olive oil and brown the fennel pieces on either side until dark golden (you may have to do this in batches, depending on the size of your dish).

4. Arrange the browned fennel pieces in a single layer in the pan and season with a little salt and pepper. Squeeze over the orange juice and pour in 75ml of water. Put the lid on and transfer to the preheated oven.

5. Braise the fennel for 25–35 minutes, until very soft but still retaining its shape. Check the dish occasionally and if the fennel looks like it is drying out, add another 75ml of water.

6. Meanwhile, for the gremolata, mix together the orange zest, parsley and garlic in a small bowl. Season with a little pinch of salt and pepper.

7. Place a frying pan over a high heat and add a little oil. When it's hot, add the duck breasts. Cook for around 12 minutes for medium. Remove the meat from the pan and allow to rest for 5 minutes.

8. Once the fennel is cooked, remove from the oven and leave to rest for 5 minutes, then serve with sliced duck breast and gremolata with any reserved fronds sprinkled on top.

PER SERVING	
KCAL	352
FAT (g)	19.0
SATURATES (g)	6.0
CARBS (g)	3.0
SUGARS (g)	3.0
FIBRE (g)	4.0
PROTEIN (g)	39.0
SALT (g)	0.4

GOOD TO KNOW
So much of the goodness in citrus fruit is in the zest, which is very fibre- and nutrient-dense, so grate it over your food whenever you can. It livens up fish, chicken, pasta, salads, dips, cocktails . . .

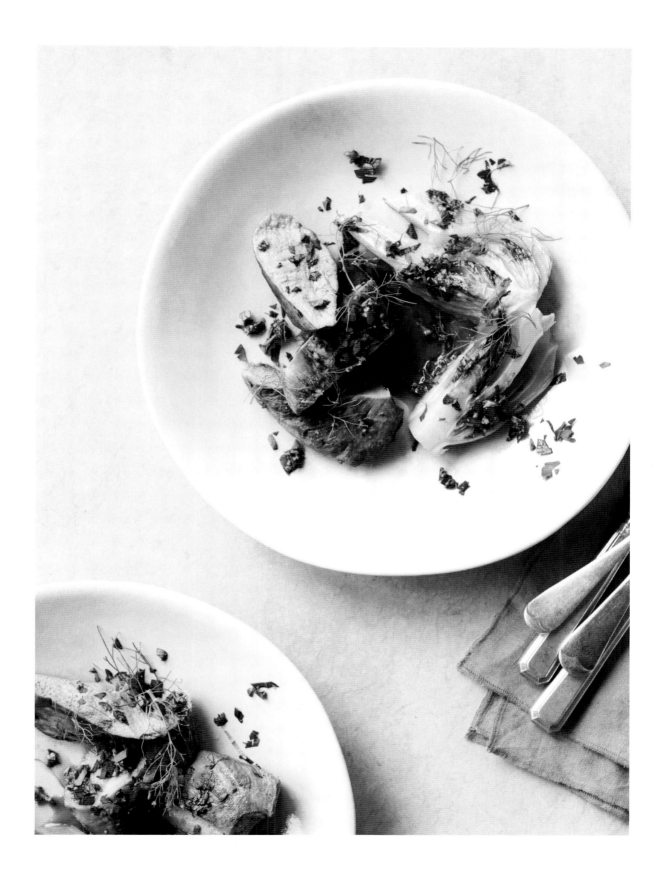

VELVETED PORK LOIN WITH GINGER SUSHI RICE AND PICKLED VEGETABLES

SERVES 2

Velveting is a Chinese cooking method that keeps meat tender when it is exposed to high temperatures. By marinating the pork in a combination of cornflour and egg white, you are literally creating a barrier that seals in the moisture that is usually lost in cooking. Velveting works particularly well with lean meats that are prone to drying out, such as chicken breasts and pork loin, but also works brilliantly with strips of beef and duck.

1 egg white
15g cornflour
20ml light soy sauce
10g honey
2 garlic cloves, peeled and finely chopped
6 cm piece of fresh root ginger, peeled
300g pork tenderloin, trimmed of sinew
    and cut into ½cm slices
50ml rice vinegar
1 tsp sugar
1 tsp fine salt
100g cucumber, deseeded, halved lengthways
    and sliced
1 red chilli, deseeded and finely sliced
80g mooli or radishes, trimmed and finely sliced
175g sushi rice
Pea shoots, to serve

PER SERVING	
KCAL	548
FAT (g)	4.0
SATURATES (g)	1.0
CARBS (g)	84.0
SUGARS (g)	8.0
FIBRE (g)	2.0
PROTEIN (g)	42.0
SALT (g)	3.07

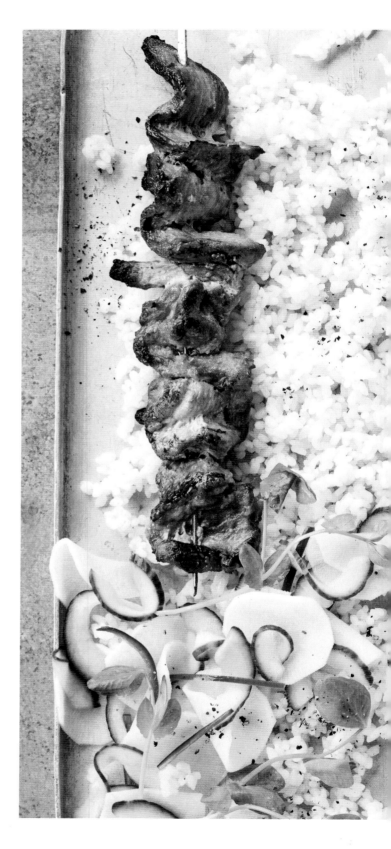

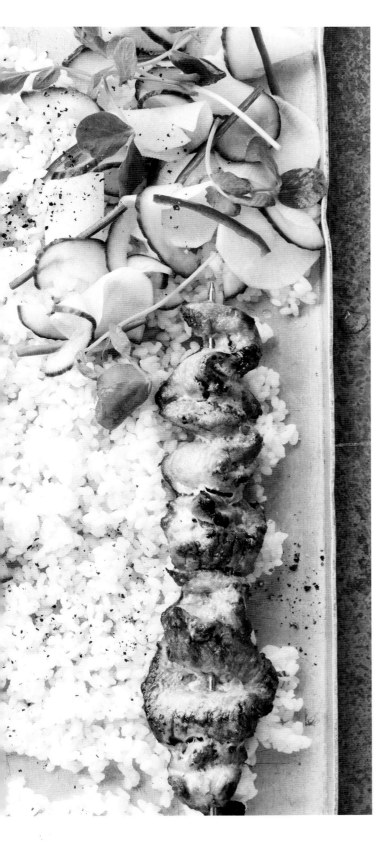

1. Whisk together the egg white, cornflour, soy sauce, honey and crushed garlic in a large bowl.

2. Grate the ginger into a sieve over a bowl, then use the back of a spoon to squeeze the juice from the ginger into the bowl. Mix the squeezed ginger flesh into the egg white mixture, then cover the ginger juice and store in the fridge until required.

3. Put the pork slices into the egg white mixture and make sure they are all well covered. Cover and leave to marinate for a minimum of 2 hours, but preferably overnight.

4. When ready to cook, mix the reserved ginger juice with the rice vinegar, sugar and salt. Tip all but 2 tablespoons of the liquid into a bowl, then add the cucumber, chilli and the mooli or radishes and toss them in the liquid. Leave the vegetables to steep for 1 hour, stirring occasionally.

5. Soak the sushi rice in cold water for 20 minutes, then strain through a sieve and rinse under cold water. Tip the rice into a small saucepan and add 175ml of water. Bring the water to the boil over a high heat, then cover with a tight lid, reduce the heat to its lowest setting and cook for 13 minutes – do not remove the lid at any point.

6. After 13 minutes, turn the heat off completely and leave the rice to stand for a minimum of 5 minutes, without removing the lid.

7. Preheat the grill to high.

8. Thread the marinated meat on to two skewers (if using bamboo skewers, soak them in water for 20 minutes beforehand). Grill for 8 minutes on one side, then flip and cook for a further 4 minutes on the second side until nicely browned and cooked through.

9. When ready to serve, remove the lid from the rice pan and pour in the remaining 2 tablespoons of ginger juice mixture. Use a fork to rough up the rice and to help it absorb the liquid.

10. Drain the pickled vegetables and serve them with the rice, pork skewers and a handful of pea shoots.

VENISON CARPACCIO
WITH CELERIAC SLAW

SERVES 4

Venison is naturally very lean and has more protein than any other red meat, making it very filling – excellent for satisfying the appetite when you are watching what you eat. It should always be served pink in the middle but I also love it raw like this, as it's meltingly tender and full of flavour. An autumnal salad with a yoghurt-based dressing like this one is the perfect garnish.

1 venison fillet (approximately 500g)
30ml rapeseed oil
25ml cider vinegar
1½ tsp Dijon mustard
50g 0% fat Greek yoghurt
1 small celeriac, peeled and julienned
1 Granny Smith apple, peeled, cored and julienned
40g walnut pieces
40g raisins
3 celery sticks, trimmed and thickly sliced diagonally
Sea salt and freshly ground black pepper

TO SERVE
Watercress
50g blackberries, halved

1. Place a large frying pan over a high heat. Brush the venison fillet all over with a little of the rapeseed oil, then season with salt and pepper.

2. When the pan is smoking hot, quickly brown the venison all over. Remove the meat from the pan and leave to cool to room temperature.

3. Lay a piece of cling film on a board and place the venison on top. Roll the venison in the cling film until you have a tight sausage shape and secure it tightly at each end. Put the venison into the fridge and leave to sit for 2 hours, or preferably overnight.

4. Just before serving, whisk together the remaining oil, cider vinegar, mustard and yoghurt with 50ml of warm water.

5. Place the julienned celeriac, apple, walnut pieces, raisins and celery in a bowl, pour over the dressing, then toss until everything is well coated.

6. Unravel the venison from the cling film and slice it as thinly as you can. Divide the slices between four plates, laying them flat in a single layer. Top with the celeriac salad and finish with a big handful of watercress and a few blackberry halves scattered over the top.

PER SERVING	
KCAL	333
FAT (g)	17.0
SATURATES (g)	2.0
CARBS (g)	11.0
SUGARS (g)	11.0
FIBRE (g)	4.0
PROTEIN (g)	32.0
SALT (g)	0.51

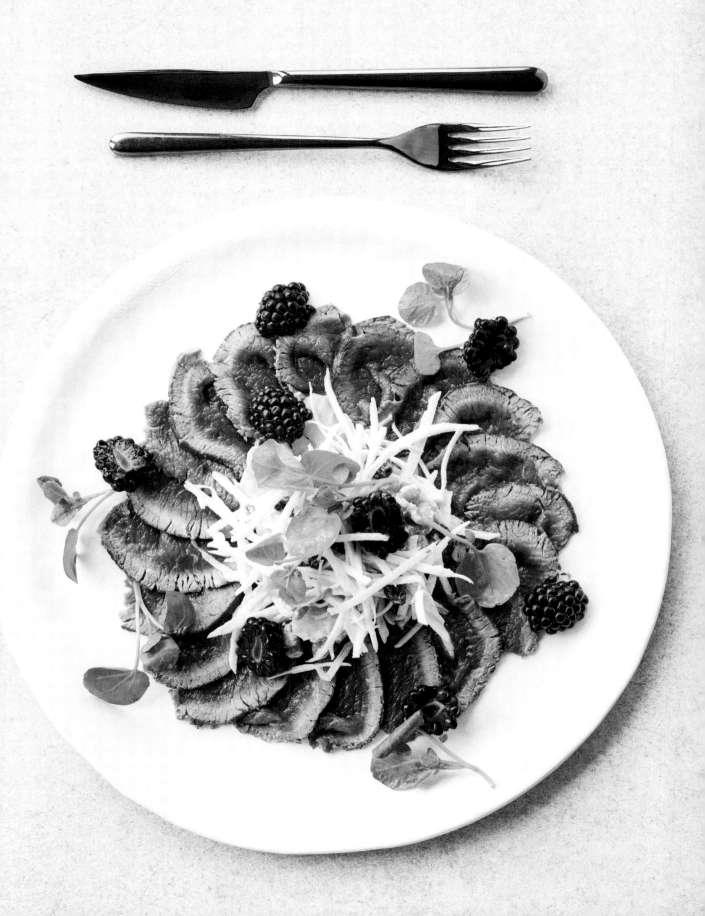

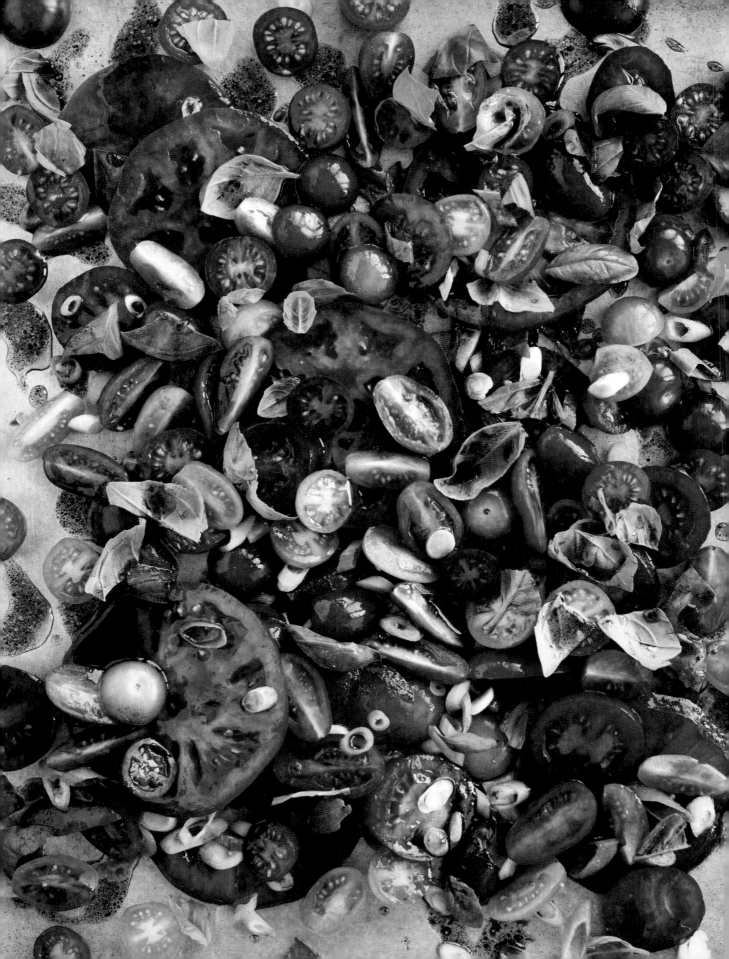

MARINATED TOMATO SALAD

SERVES 4 AS A SIDE

Marinating tomatoes for a couple of hours before you eat them totally transforms a regular tomato salad into a sensational one. Trust me, it's really worth doing. The flavours really intensify, as does the nutrient content, and the tomatoes come alive. Choose ripe tomatoes of different colours and sizes, and use a really good-quality extra virgin olive oil – it will make all the difference.

1kg ripe tomatoes
3 spring onions or 1 small shallot,
   very finely diced
Small bunch of basil, leaves only
1½ tbsp balsamic or sherry vinegar
4 tbsp extra virgin olive oil
Sea salt and freshly ground black pepper

1. Slice, halve or quarter the tomatoes, depending on their size, and put them all into a large serving bowl.

2. Sprinkle over the spring onions or diced shallot, then tear the basil leaves and add them on top.

3. Pour in the vinegar and olive oil and add a good pinch of salt and pepper, then, using your hands, gently mix these through the tomatoes, taking care not to bruise any of the ripe fruit.

4. Cover the dish and leave at room temperature for 1 hour or up to 3 hours before serving.

PER SERVING	
KCAL	149
FAT (g)	11.0
SATURATES (g)	2.0
CARBS (g)	9.0
SUGARS (g)	8.0
FIBRE (g)	3.0
PROTEIN (g)	2.0
SALT (g)	0.02

GUILT-FREE TREATS

ICED GREEN TEA

SERVES 4

Iced tea is hugely popular in America, and in health-conscious California it is green tea with all its antioxidants, flavonoids and polyphenols (phytochemicals valued for their protective properties) that is iced even more than black tea. Make a big jugful and sip it through the day to keep you hydrated and take your mind off sugary snacks at the same time.

4 green tea teabags
Runny honey, to taste
1 unwaxed lemon, sliced

1. Put the teabags into a heatproof container such as a large teapot or jug. Pour over 1.25 litres of just-boiled water and sweeten with runny honey (approx. 1–1½ tablespoons) to taste.

2. Add the lemon slices and leave to steep until cool, then remove the teabags.

3. Taste and add more honey if necessary.

4. Serve in tall glasses with lots of ice.

PER SERVING	
KCAL	23
FAT (g)	0.1
SATURATES (g)	0.0
CARBS (g)	5.0
SUGARS (g)	4.0
FIBRE (g)	0.5
PROTEIN (g)	1.0
SALT (g)	0.01

VARIATIONS
You can add different flavours to this tea – slices of fresh root ginger or lime are brilliant to add during the steeping process, as are sprigs of herbs such as mint or lemon thyme, or even metabolism-boosting spices like cayenne and chilli.

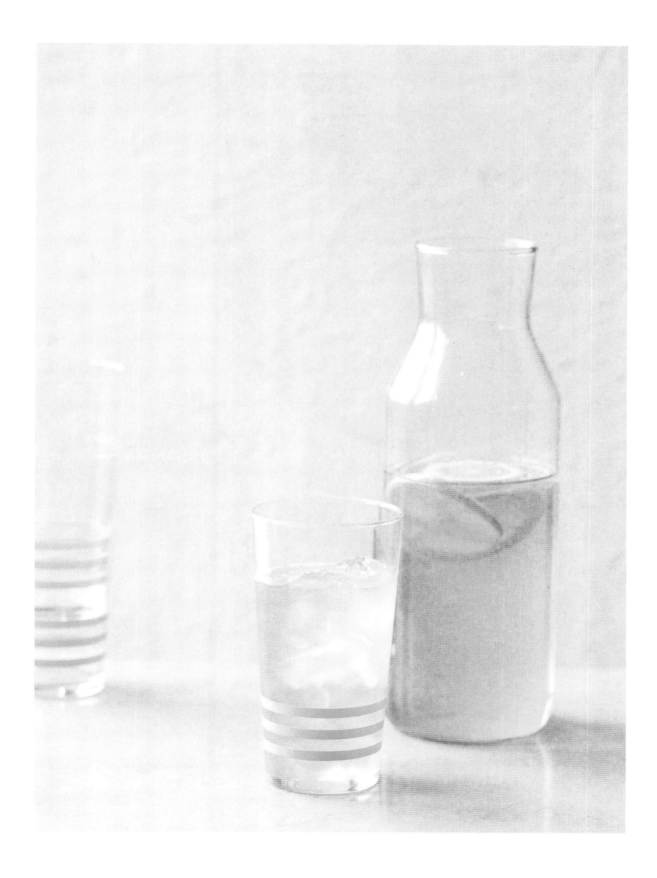

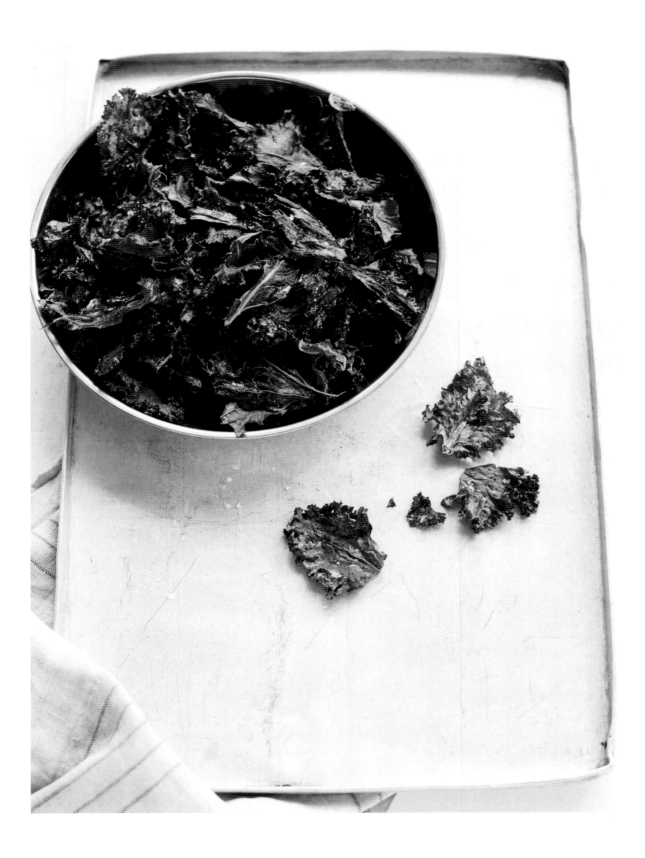

MAPLE SOY KALE CRISPS

SERVES 4

Roasting kale in this way changes it from a raw cabbage leaf into a crisp snack that tastes like the crispy seaweed you get in Chinese restaurants but is much better for you. Kale crisps are also delicious crumbled over salads or sprinkled over Asian dishes, giving them an intense, salty hit.

200g kale or cavolo nero leaves, stalks removed, washed and dried
1 tbsp maple syrup
1 tbsp olive oil
1 tsp soy sauce
Pinch of salt

1. Preheat the oven to 150°C/gas 2.

2. Slice the kale into bite-sized pieces the same size as potato crisps.

3. Put the maple syrup, olive oil, soy sauce and a pinch of salt into a large bowl and mix together. Add the kale to the bowl and massage the marinade into the leaves, making sure that every piece of kale is coated.

4. Spread the kale in a single layer on one or two baking trays. Put the trays into the preheated oven and bake for 7–10 minutes. After 5 minutes, check the kale and swap the trays over if using more than one tray. Continue to cook until the kale is crisp but not burning. Some pieces may cook faster than others, in which case remove the pieces that are crisp and continue to cook the remaining pieces until they are also crisp. Leave to cool.

5. Once cool, they can be stored in an airtight container for up to a week.

VARIATIONS
Kale crisps are a great vehicle for lots of different flavours, such as chilli, lime, wasabi or Parmesan cheese. For paprika crisps, follow the method above but marinate the kale in 1 tbsp olive oil, 1 tsp smoked paprika, ½ tsp garlic granules, 1 tsp chilli flakes (optional) and a pinch of salt.

PER SERVING	
KCAL	59
FAT (g)	4.0
SATURATES (g)	1.0
CARBS (g)	4.0
SUGARS (g)	4.0
FIBRE (g)	2.0
PROTEIN (g)	2.0
SALT (g)	0.23

SMOKY SPICED POPCORN

SERVES 4

Making your own popcorn is really easy and, if you keep the amount of oil down, much better for you than commercial brands, which can be just as fattening per 100g as potato crisps. Spicing up your popcorn is a clever way to help you eat less of it, too. This combination of sweet, smoky paprika and warming garam masala is amazing, but you could also experiment with other favourite spices like cinnamon, cumin or black pepper.

2 tbsp sunflower oil
100g popcorn kernels
Pinch of salt
1 tsp sweet smoked paprika
½ tsp garam masala

1. Place a large saucepan with a tight-fitting lid over a medium–high heat and add the oil.

2 When the oil is very hot (see below), sprinkle in the popcorn kernels and put the lid on. Once you hear the kernels start to pop, give the pan a little shake approximately every 30 seconds. When the sound of the corn popping has died down, turn off the heat and carefully remove the lid.

3. Put the salt, paprika and garam masala into a small bowl and mix together until thoroughly blended.

4. Tip the popcorn into a large tray and sprinkle with the spiced salt, tossing gently until coated evenly. Eat immediately, or keep in an airtight container for a couple of days.

PER SERVING	
KCAL	141
FAT (g)	7.0
SATURATES (g)	1.0
CARBS (g)	15.0
SUGARS (g)	0.3
FIBRE (g)	3.0
PROTEIN (g)	3.0
SALT (g)	0.37

HOW TO MAKE POPCORN
A clever way of telling when the oil is hot enough before adding the popcorn is to add three kernels first. When all three of them have popped, the oil is ready to go.

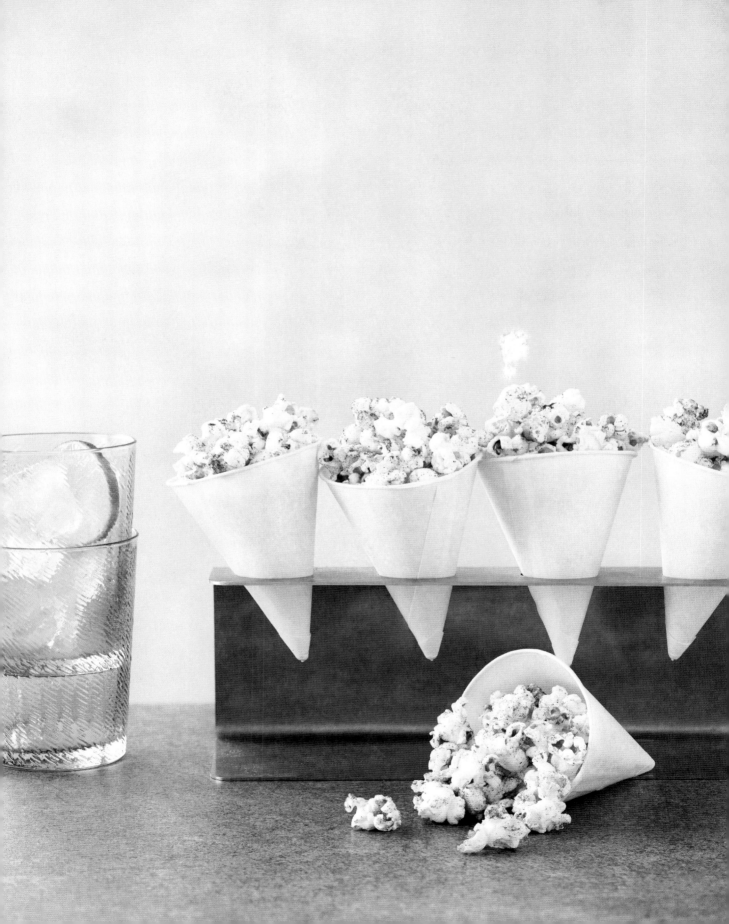

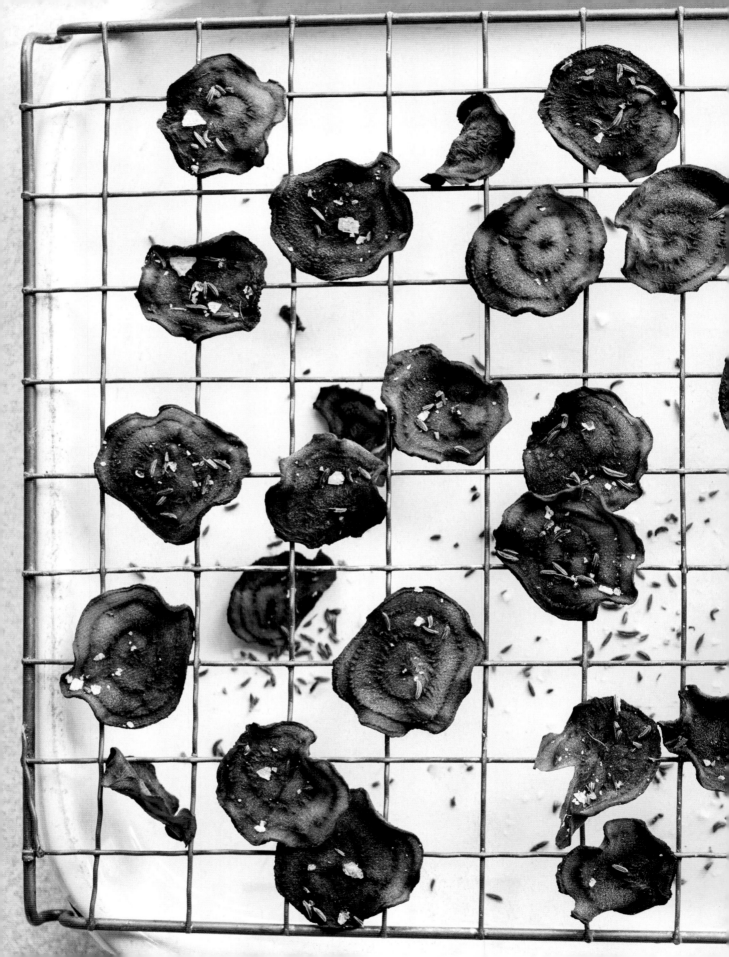

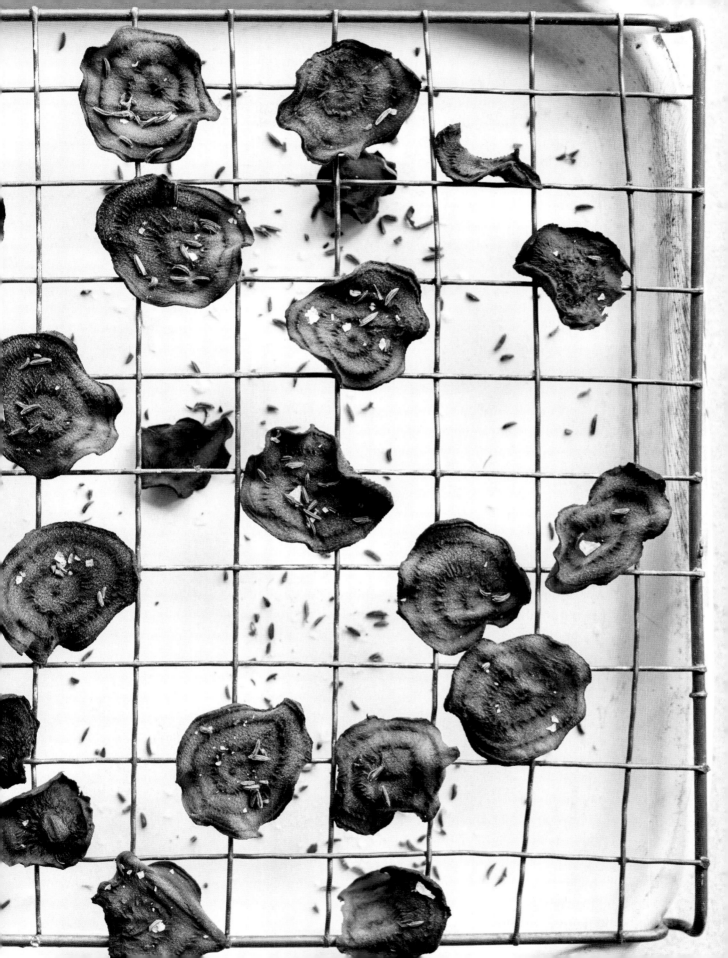

CARAWAY BEETROOT CRISPS

SERVES 4

Traditional crisps are off the menu when you are trying to lose weight because they are so high in fat and because we tend to eat more than we should once we start, but these healthy beetroot crisps are fat- and guilt-free, so you can eat as many as you like and they make a contribution to your five-a-day. They go brilliantly with dips like Baba Ganoush (see page 95) and Houmous (see page 94). If you don't eat them all in one sitting, the crisps will keep in an airtight container for up to two days.

3 medium beetroot (approximately 330g), peeled
2 tsp caraway seeds, toasted
1 tsp sea salt

1. Preheat the oven to 160°C/gas 3.

2. Place two cooling racks on top of two baking trays. If you don't have cooling racks, use baking trays lined with greaseproof paper. (This will take longer, so don't remove the beetroot from the oven until it's definitely crisp.)

3. Finely slice the beetroots, ideally with a mandolin or a very sharp knife.

4. Lay the slices out in a thin layer on the racks, trying not to let them overlap. Bake the slices in the preheated oven for 15–20 minutes.

5. Meanwhile, crush the toasted caraway seeds and sea salt together in a pestle and mortar.

6. After 15 minutes, check the crisps and if they're not quite crisp continue to cook for longer – the time will depend on how thick the beetroot slices are.

7. When the crisps have finished cooking, remove the trays from the oven and leave them to cool on the racks.

8. When cool, transfer the crisps to a bowl and sprinkle with the caraway salt, carefully tossing them to ensure an even coating.

PER SERVING	
KCAL	38
FAT (g)	0.3
SATURATES (g)	0.0
CARBS (g)	6.0
SUGARS (g)	5.0
FIBRE (g)	2.0
PROTEIN (g)	2.0
SALT (g)	1.36

SPICED APPLE SORBET

SERVES 4

Sorbet is much lighter than ice cream in terms of fat content but it's still packed with flavour, which makes this the perfect sweet hit for the end of a meal, particularly in autumn when apples are at their best. By choosing red apples the sorbet will have a hint of pink from the skins, which makes it very pretty as well as refreshing – a perfect palate cleanser.

6 medium red-skinned apples, quartered and cored
1 tbsp maple syrup
Juice of 1 lemon
2 tsp ground cinnamon
½ tsp ground cardamom
1 tsp ground ginger

1. Chop the apples into chunks and put them into a saucepan with the maple syrup, 250ml of water, the lemon juice, cinnamon, cardamom and ginger. Bring to a simmer over a medium–low heat, stirring often, until the apples have completely collapsed and an apple purée has formed.

2. Taste the mixture and add a little more maple syrup if needed, remembering that when the mixture is frozen the flavours will be dulled slightly so any sweetness or sourness will not be so pronounced.

3. Pour into a food processor and blend until completely smooth.

4. Put the mixture into a freezer-safe container with a lid and freeze for at least 6 hours, or until set.

5. Remove the sorbet from the freezer 15 minutes before serving to soften slightly.

PER SERVING	
KCAL	98
FAT (g)	1.0
SATURATES (g)	0.2
CARBS (g)	20.0
SUGARS (g)	20.0
FIBRE (g)	3.0
PROTEIN (g)	1.0
SALT (g)	0.01

BANANA 'ICE CREAM'

SERVES 4

My daughter Tilly introduced me to this genius recipe . . . it's a one-ingredient, dairy-free, fat-free ice cream with no added sugar that you don't need an ice cream machine to make – it's incredible! You can add all sorts of things to the base recipe, like peanut butter, frozen berries, chocolate chips, cocoa nibs, coconut flakes or chopped nuts (see page 277 for a coconut and chocolate version). Just make sure you don't add any liquid or it will lose its ice cream-like consistency.

4 ripe bananas, peeled

1. Slice the banana into chunks and put them into a freezer-proof container. Put the container into the freezer and leave overnight or until frozen solid.

2. When ready to make the ice cream, put the frozen banana pieces into a food processor and pulse to break them up into small pieces. Scrape down the sides of the food processor, then blend until the banana is smooth and creamy, stopping regularly to scrape down the sides.

3. Eat immediately for a soft-serve consistency or put it back into a freezer-proof container and freeze for 1 hour until hard.

PER SERVING	
KCAL	86
FAT (g)	0.1
SATURATES (g)	0.0
CARBS (g)	19.0
SUGARS (g)	17.0
FIBRE (g)	1.0
PROTEIN (g)	1.0
SALT (g)	0.04

COCONUT ICE LOLLIES

MAKES 6 LOLLIES

This is another excellent dairy-free ice cream that doesn't need an ice cream machine. You can make it without the fruit, as the coconut has such a delicious flavour on its own, or stir through some desiccated coconut and lime zest for extra texture and bite. This is the kind of guilt-free indulgence that really helps to keep you on track when willpower is beginning to weaken.

200ml coconut milk
1 tbsp maple syrup
100g fresh or frozen fruit, e.g. blueberries, raspberries or mango chunks

1. Put the coconut milk and maple syrup into a jug and mix until completely combined. Stir in the fruit.

2. Divide the mixture between the lolly moulds.

3. Put lolly sticks into the moulds and transfer to the freezer for at least 4 hours but ideally overnight.

4. To serve, remove from the freezer and allow to warm slightly before trying to pull the lollies out of the moulds.

VARIATIONS
They are great made with blueberries, raspberries, blackberries or mango, all of which freeze really well. Keep bags of frozen fruits in the freezer so you can make these ice lollies all year round even if your fruit bowl is empty.

PER SERVING	
KCAL	71
FAT (g)	6.0
SATURATES (g)	5.0
CARBS (g)	4.0
SUGARS (g)	3.0
FIBRE (g)	1.0
PROTEIN (g)	1.0
SALT (g)	0.01

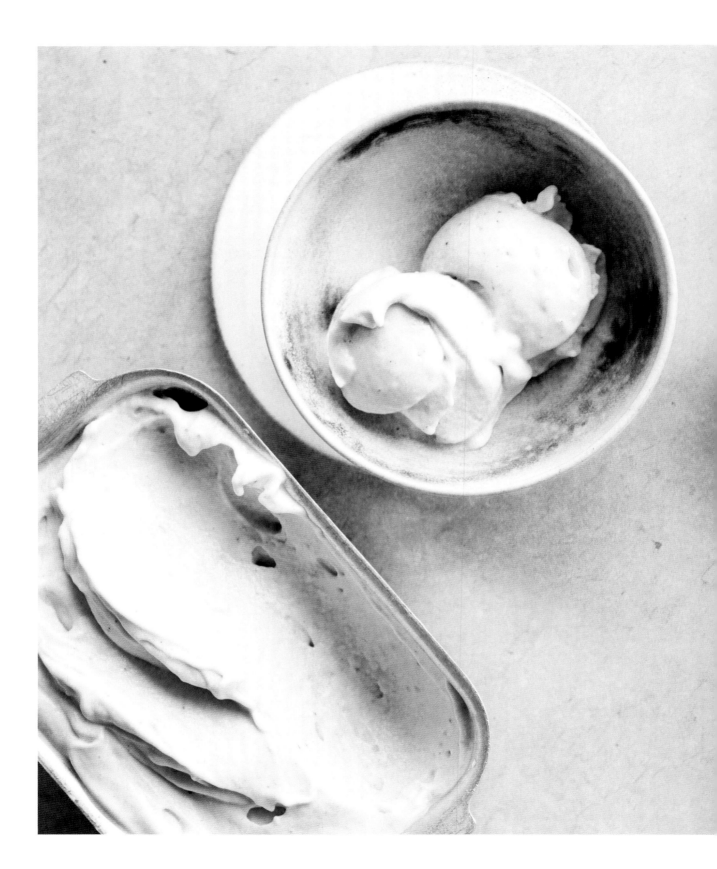

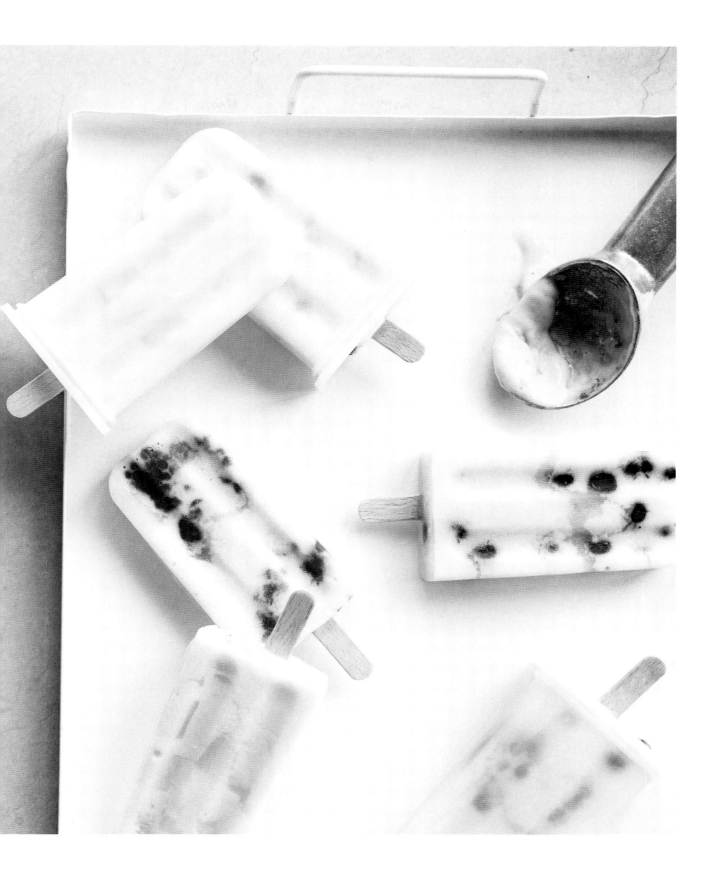

CARROT CAKE MACAROONS

MAKES 18 MACAROONS

These macaroons are not to be muddled up with French macarons, which are those delicate meringue spaceships that are full of sugar and can be a bit tricky to cook outside a professional pastry kitchen. These are the coconut macaroons of my childhood, updated to taste a lot like carrot cake but without all that butter icing. When cake is off the menu, have a couple of these to keep the sweet cravings at bay.

200g unsweetened desiccated coconut
1½ tsp ground cinnamon
1 tsp ground ginger
½ tsp freshly grated nutmeg
50g walnuts, chopped
1 large carrot, grated
75g golden caster sugar
4 egg whites
Pinch of salt

1. Preheat the oven to 170°C/gas 3.

2. Put the coconut, cinnamon, ginger and nutmeg into a bowl and mix well.

3. Add the chopped walnuts, grated carrot, sugar, egg whites and a pinch of salt and mix together until everything is fully incorporated.

4. Line a baking tray with greaseproof paper and drop 18–20 heaped dessertspoons of the mixture on to the tray, leaving a gap of at least 1cm between them. Shape the mounds so that they are roughly circular.

5. Put the tray into the preheated oven and bake for 15–20 minutes, until golden and firm on the outside. Leave to cool on a wire rack before serving.

PER MACAROON	
KCAL	115
FAT (g)	9.0
SATURATES (g)	6.0
CARBS (g)	5.0
SUGARS (g)	5.0
FIBRE (g)	2.0
PROTEIN (g)	2.0
SALT (g)	0.05

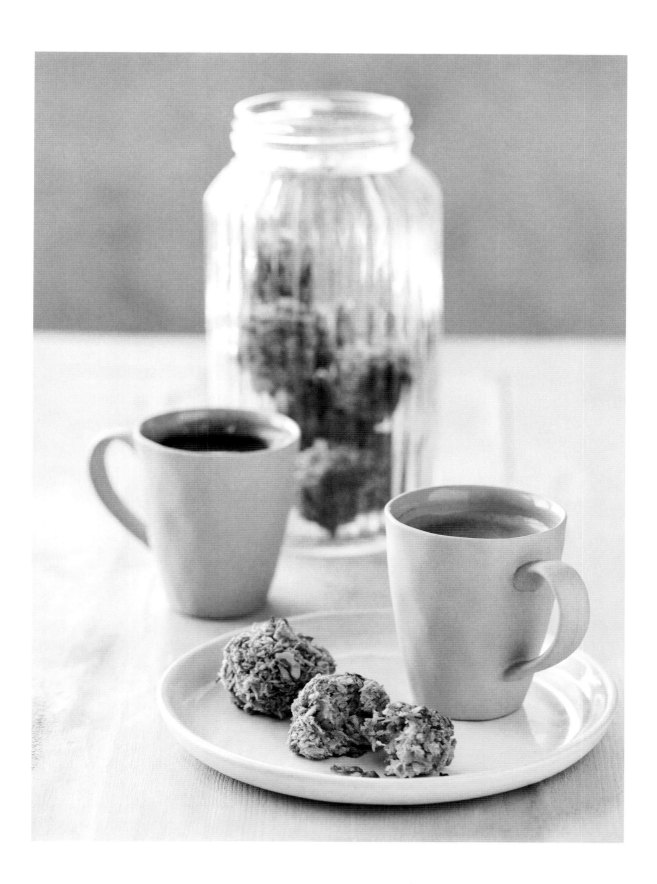

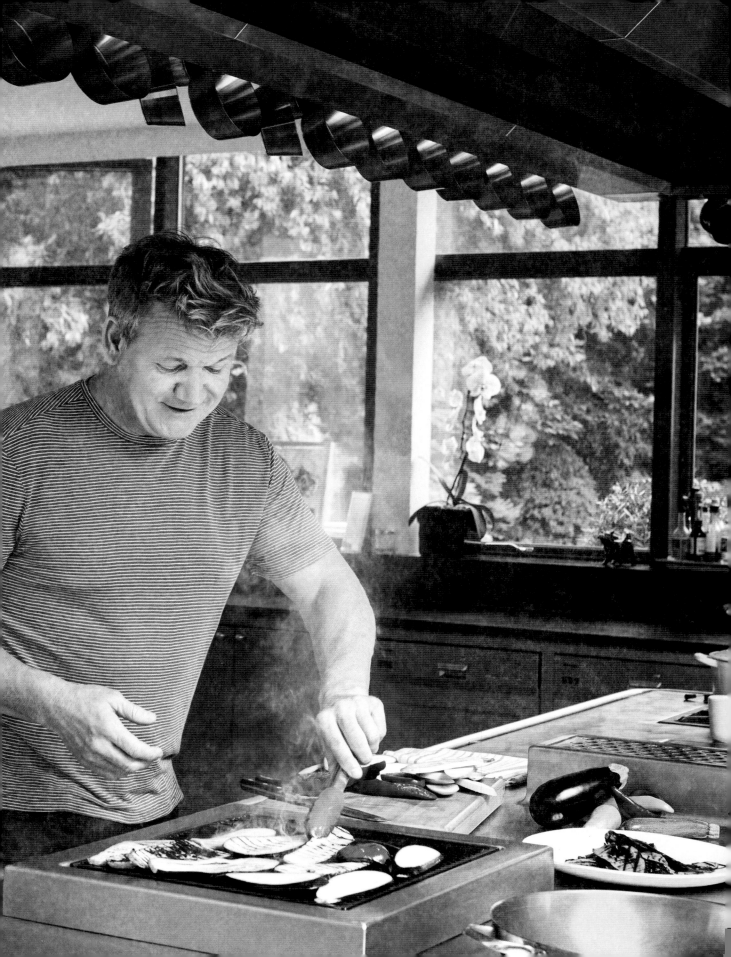

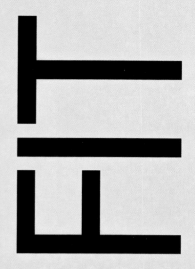

TAKING EXERCISE IS COMPLETELY ESSENTIAL FOR MY WELLBEING

Wherever I am in the world, I find a way to fit in a workout, run or swim, often as soon as I arrive in a new city. It is my release from a very busy schedule and it helps me deal with the pressures I face. To keep myself fit and motivated, I always sign up for two major races a year and when I'm not injured, I try to train properly at least three times a week, usually first thing in the morning, then I go for a huge bike ride on Sundays, sometimes with Tana or my son Jack. So far, I have run 15 marathons, three ultramarathons, four half Ironmans (a triathlon followed by a half marathon) and the world's toughest Ironman in Hawaii. And it's not just me – Tana has run seven marathons and two half Ironmans, too, and my daughter Megan has just competed in her first marathon at just 18!

Given that I am almost always in training for something, I always have to keep an eye on the food I consume. Happily, my eating habits as a chef are quite similar to those recommended for athletes and sportsmen – eating little and often, which stabilizes blood sugar and keeps energy levels topped up, and not over-eating, which slows the body down. When I'm training, I have to spend more time trying to get the right balance of carbohydrates, proteins and fats needed for endurance. Fuel is just so important for performance – it not only helps you operate to the best of your abilities, it also reduces the risk of illness and injury and aids post-exercise recovery. If you aren't eating the right foods or getting enough liquids to keep you hydrated, you will struggle with fatigue, weakness and may even pick up strains and sprains.

Though each sport and each individual sportsman or woman requires a slightly different combination of macronutrients to deliver the best results, there are a few general rules involving what to eat and when to eat it that apply to everyone. To put it simply, it's really important to get enough carbohydrates before you do any exercise, and equally important to follow up a tough session with some lean protein for muscle repair and some more carbs to restock your energy levels. It's also essential that you drink enough water – becoming dehydrated will not only hinder your performance, it can be seriously bad for your health.

Understanding a bit more about basic sports nutrition and how the body works will help you prepare yourself for exercise challenges and maybe even improve your personal best! In this section, you will find recipes that have been designed to help you get the right balance of macronutrients when you need them and, given that they are some of my personal training favourites, they taste really good too. The recipes here are sometimes higher in calories than in the previous two sections because they assume a very active lifestyle. And by active, I don't mean a water aerobics class once a week! This is food for training and endurance sessions that last at least an hour and much longer.

CARB-LOADING

One of the key components of eating right for sports and training is the increased intake of carbohydrates before a big match or race. This is known as carb-loading and it is essential for fuelling your muscles so they can deliver on the day. But how does it work? Putting it simply, when you eat carbs, they are broken down by the body to form glucose, which provides readily available energy for the body to use. Any extra glucose is stored in the muscles and liver in the form of glycogen for when the body needs it. Basically, glycogen is the reserve fuel that drives your muscles.

Because the body can only store a certain amount of glycogen at a time, it's important to keep topping the levels up, particularly before exercise. If you don't, you will tire easily, lack power and under-perform. Normally, carbohydrates should make up about a third of every meal, but this amount needs to increase as your exercise levels increase. And during the day or two before and on the morning of a big event, carb intake should rise to more than three-quarters of your food consumption.

Typically, the best carbohydrates to choose for exercise are the complex, unrefined varieties, which take longer for the body to break down and therefore release their energy more slowly. Good choices include wholemeal bread, porridge oats, brown pasta, noodles, brown rice, couscous, potatoes, parsnips, sweetcorn, peas, sweet potatoes, lentils, beans and fruit. As you get closer to race day, however, you can eat more refined carbs like white rice, pasta, bagels and white bread, because they are so easy to digest and will lay down plenty of energy for physical exertion. It can feel quite repetitive and dull to eat pasta every night so I make sure I vary the carbs I eat and serve them with punchy sauces and strong flavours to keep it interesting. (See page 226 for a chef's recipes for carb-loading.)

Most people start carb-loading a few days before a big race but I like to start increasing my carb intake about six weeks in advance. It helps you to work out which carbs suit you in larger quantities and which ones don't, and it gets your body used to the increased carb levels. And with the increased glycogen levels, your training will be much more effective, too. Then, three or four days before the race, you should increase your intake further until it is making up 85–90% of your plate. Choose meals from the carb-loading chapter in this section for the eve of a race or event, then have a carb-rich breakfast early in the morning of the big day to further maximize your glycogen levels. For a final top-up, you should have an energy-charged snack at least 30 minutes before the start – less than 30 minutes and your body will still be digesting it when the starting gun sounds. Carb-loading in this way will ensure that you have the energy you need to get through the trial ahead, and I can't stress enough how important it is to get it right. Not having enough fuel in the tank can lead to low blood sugar, dizziness and extreme exhaustion, otherwise known as 'hitting the wall', and you will find yourself crashing out of the race.

RECOVERY

When it's all over and you are exhausted, elated and aching all over, it is vital to eat or drink some form of protein, ideally within 30 minutes of finishing. Protein is needed for the repair and growth of muscles and, given that you have just put yours under incredible stress, they will need some TLC. Getting some protein in quickly will stop your muscles from being too sore (though they will still ache!) and help you to recover more quickly.

To maximize the efficiency of the protein, it's important to keep the amount of fat down because it can slow the uptake of the protein when you need it quickly. Therefore, choose lean sources like eggs, dairy products and lean meat. A milkshake is ideal because not only does it supply protein and carbs, it also rehydrates the body at the same time and is easy to get your head around straight after exercising, when you might not fancy a chicken sandwich. You need to keep eating protein for 24 hours after a big race, so pick one of the high-protein meals in the recovery section for your celebration feast – just make sure you get someone else to cook it while you have a well-deserved rest!

You also need yet more carbohydrate after exercise to refuel the glycogen levels in your muscles and again, at this point, it's OK to have fast-acting simple carbs which can be digested quickly and easily. You need to drink plenty of fluid too, to replace all the liquid lost through sweat and to avoid dehydration. And then rest . . . most muscle reparation happens while you are sleeping, so go to bed early and let your body do all the hard work.

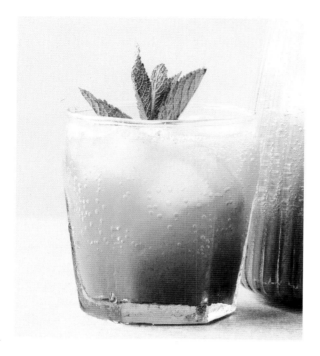

HYDRATION FOR SPORTS

Drinking plenty of liquid is essential for good health but even more important when you are training and pushing yourself physically. Becoming dehydrated can seriously affect your performance, so make sure you take in plenty of liquid in advance. About two hours before a race, drink approximately 500ml of water, diluted fruit juice or a sports drink, and drink another 150ml of fluid 30 minutes before you start. This should allow your body to get rid of any liquid it doesn't need before you get going. Drink small amounts while running to keep levels topped up as you sweat, and make sure you drink plenty of fluid afterwards to get back to normal hydration levels. Also, be aware that different climates, seasons, altitudes and weather can affect how much water you need, so do some research in advance and be prepared. Getting enough liquid for your body's needs will make all the difference on the day.

ACTIVE KIDS

My four children are all really sporty. As I mentioned, my oldest daughter, Megan, has just run her first marathon aged 18 and it can be hard to keep track of the different sports the rest of them play – water polo, netball, lacrosse, hockey, athletics, etc. They're all really keen on running, cycling and swimming, too, and though I'm not sure whether it's genetic or purely driven by Tana and me, you would definitely say we're a pretty active family.

Getting the right nutrition matters even more for active kids and teenagers because they haven't finished growing yet. It is vital that they get enough energy from the food they eat, to fuel activity, and a wide variety of micronutrients, to keep them healthy. Make sure you provide carb-based meals for supper and breakfast on match days and have plenty of energy-boosting snacks like muesli bars or Fig Rolls (see page 274) available for when they're needed. As with adults, protein is essential for muscle recovery, so encourage your kids to eat snacks like cheese, yoghurt or peanut butter sandwiches when it's all over.

It's particularly important that young people drink enough liquid before, during and after exercise, because they can get dehydrated faster than adults doing the same amount of activity. Make sure they have access to plenty of water, diluted fruit juice or low-fat milk, and encourage them to keep drinking, because children aren't always very good at monitoring their own hydration levels. With the right fuel, they will hopefully enjoy sport and exercise more and grow to be active and healthy adults with good habits for life.

BOOSTING BREAKFASTS

BANANA AND DATE BREAKFAST SHAKE

SERVES 3

A shot of slow-releasing energy from dates and bananas is a smart way to support your energy levels for a big run or competition. And a smoothie is great if you don't want to feel over-full but still want to get in the maximum amount of carbs while hydrating at the same time. I add some ice to a Thermos flask and take this shake with me for an energy boost on the go.

2 ripe bananas
8 dates (5 if using medjool dates), pitted
500ml almond milk

1. Break the bananas into chunks and put them into a blender with the dates and almond milk.

2. Blend on a high speed until smooth. For an extra cold shake, add a couple of ice cubes to the blender and blitz again.

3. Pour into 3 glasses to serve.

PER SERVING	
KCAL	196
FAT (g)	2.0
SATURATES (g)	0.2
CARBS (g)	40.0
SUGARS (g)	38.0
FIBRE (g)	4.0
PROTEIN (g)	2.0
SALT (g)	0.21

VARIATIONS
Add 1 tablespoon of cacao nibs for a chocolate hit and an injection of heart-healthy antioxidants. Swap the almond milk for cow's milk or yoghurt if you want to up your protein levels post exercise.

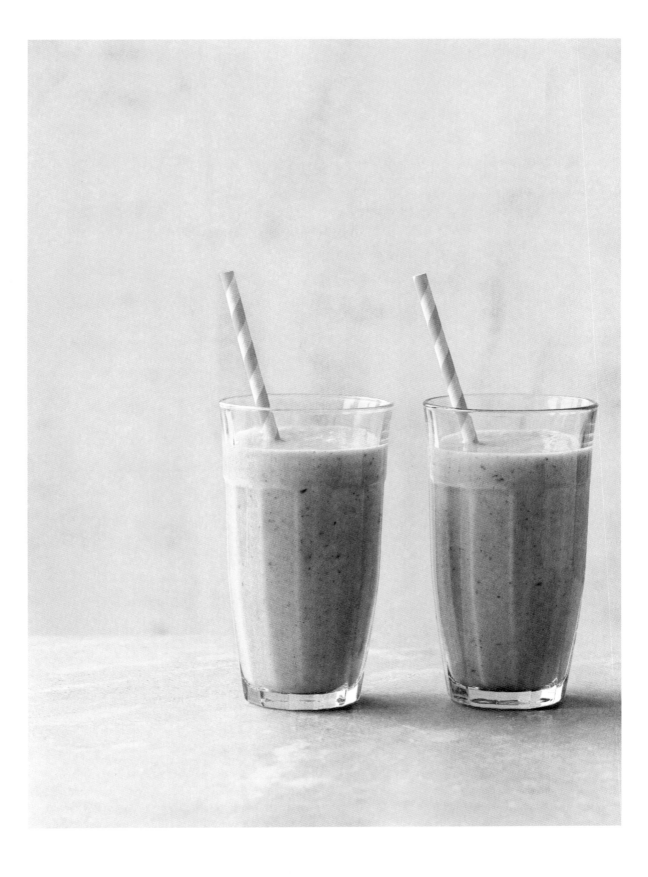

FROZEN BERRY BREAKFAST BOWL

SERVES 4

The ladies in my life love a bowl of berries like this in the morning. I think it's because it tastes a lot like ice cream! Acai berries are one of the latest superfoods to reach our shores from South America and, among the many wondrous claims made of them, they are said to boost energy levels. So, no more excuses for staying in bed . . .

6 tbsp acai juice or 4 tbsp acai powder
300g frozen berries, such as blueberries, raspberries, strawberries or mixed berries
4 bananas, peeled, broken into pieces and frozen for at least 2 hours
Water, coconut water or apple juice, if needed
1 fresh banana
4 small handfuls of granola
2 handfuls of fresh blueberries

1. Put the acai juice or powder, frozen berries and frozen bananas into a food processor or blender and blend until smooth. If the mixture looks like it needs some help blending, add a small amount of liquid, a little at a time, to get it going. The mixture should blend to a soft-serve ice cream consistency rather than a smoothie consistency.

2. Transfer to serving bowls and top with sliced fresh banana, granola and fresh blueberries. Serve immediately, before it starts to melt!

PER SERVING	
KCAL	332
FAT (g)	12.0
SATURATES (g)	4.0
CARBS (g)	43.0
SUGARS (g)	33.0
FIBRE (g)	10.0
PROTEIN (g)	7.0
SALT (g)	0.04

TO MAKE IT LEAN
Leave out the acai juice or powder and replace it with an extra 100g of frozen berries if you're watching your weight.

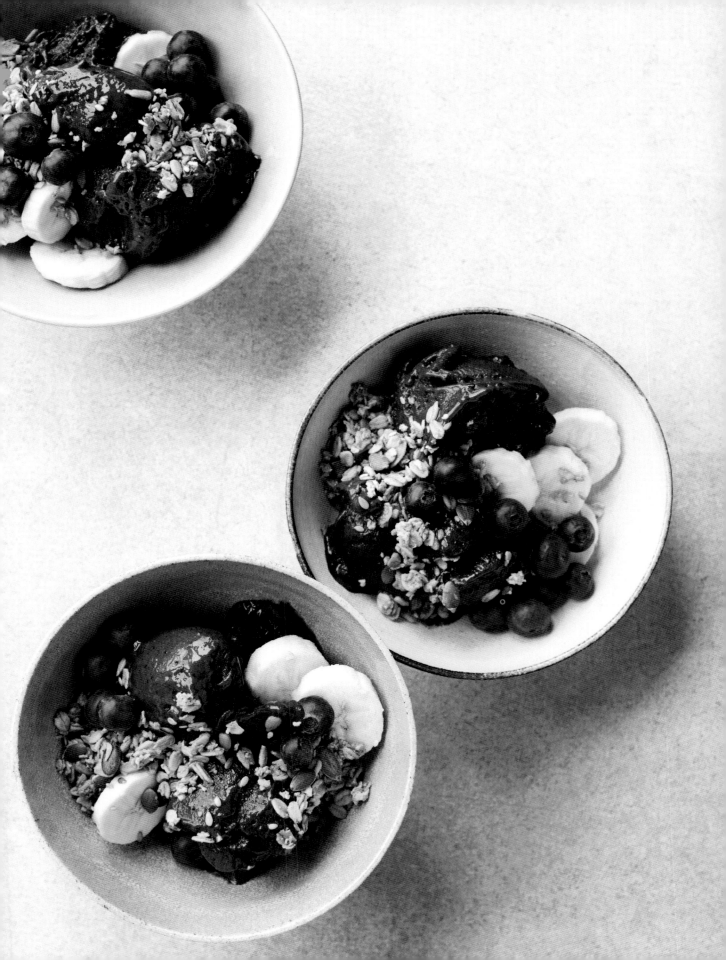

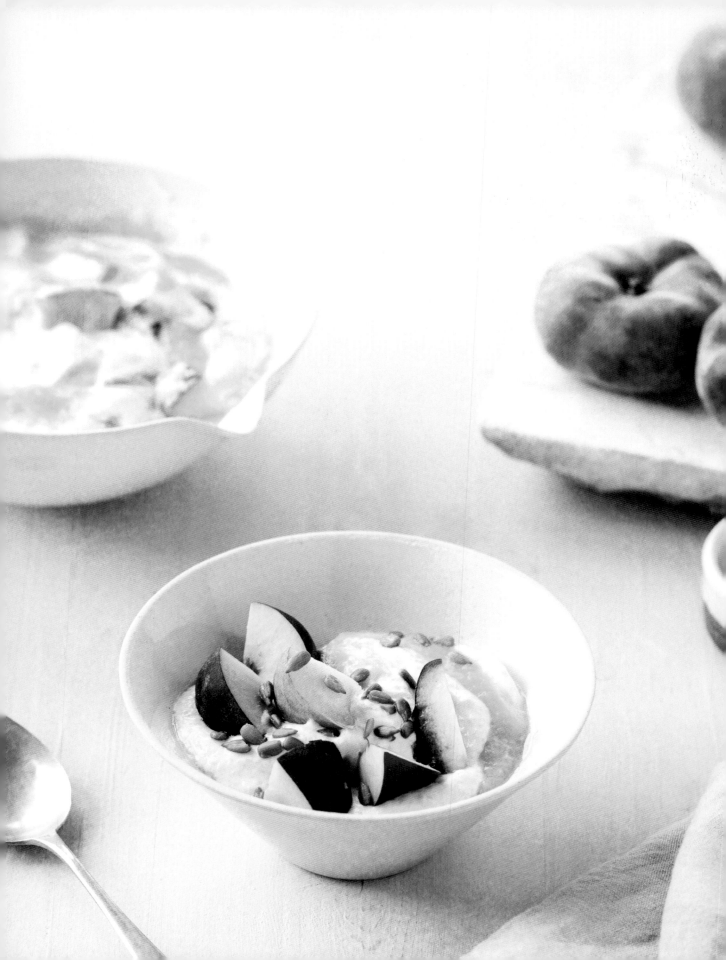

YOGHURT AND PEACH BOWL

SERVES 4

This is a really simple breakfast for the summer months, when peaches and nectarines are at their finest. The naturally occurring sugars in the fruit and honey are easily accessed and stored by the body for exertion in the day ahead, while the protein-rich yoghurt helps stabilize energy levels so you don't have a sugar crash. You can use other fruits like plums or cherries, but avoid pineapple and kiwi as they will make the yoghurt split.

8 ripe peaches or nectarines, stoned
750g natural or Greek yoghurt
2 tbsp sunflower seeds

1. Peel 4 of the peaches and chop into chunks. Place the peaches into a blender and blitz until smooth, then set aside.

2. Swirl the peach purée through the yoghurt to create a ripple effect. Cut the remaining peaches into bite-sized pieces and stir half through the peach yoghurt mixture (do not blend). Divide the yoghurt between four bowls.

3. Top each bowl with the remaining peach chunks and sprinkle the sunflower seeds over the top.

FOR EXTRA ENERGY
Sprinkle a handful of granola over the top of each bowl if you want to maximize your glycogen levels.

PER SERVING	
KCAL	350
FAT (g)	23.0
SATURATES (g)	13.0
CARBS (g)	20.0
SUGARS (g)	18.0
FIBRE (g)	3.0
PROTEIN (g)	14.0
SALT (g)	0.31

PEANUT BUTTER AND RASPBERRY JAM PANCAKES

SERVES 6

This is a simple gluten-free pancake recipe that
provides lots of energy but won't slow you down.
Make a big batch for the team and watch everyone
devour them, knowing that they will be full of good
things to draw on in the day ahead. It works just
as well with other nut butters, so swap in cashew,
hazelnut or almond butter for a change.

250g peanut butter, smooth or crunchy
5 eggs
4 tbsp natural yoghurt
3 tbsp Raspberry Chia Seed Jam (see page 32),
    plus extra for serving
1 tbsp rapeseed oil, for frying
4 bananas, peeled and sliced
Maple syrup, to serve (optional)

1. Mix the peanut butter, eggs, yoghurt and raspberry
jam together in a bowl until well combined. The
mixture should be a thick dropping consistency.

2. Place a large frying pan over a medium heat.
Add the rapeseed oil and heat, swirling around the
pan to coat. Add a heaped tablespoon of the mixture
to the pan and spread until it is the thickness of a
Scotch pancake. Cook for 2–3 minutes, until lightly
coloured, then turn over and repeat on the other side.

3. Keep the pancakes warm in a low oven or wrapped
in a tea towel while you cook the rest of the mixture.

4. Serve with the sliced banana and extra dollops
of jam, as well as a drizzle of maple syrup, if desired.

PER SERVING	
KCAL	418
FAT (g)	29.0
SATURATES (g)	7.0
CARBS (g)	18.0
SUGARS (g)	14.0
FIBRE (g)	4.0
PROTEIN (g)	19.0
SALT (g)	0.60

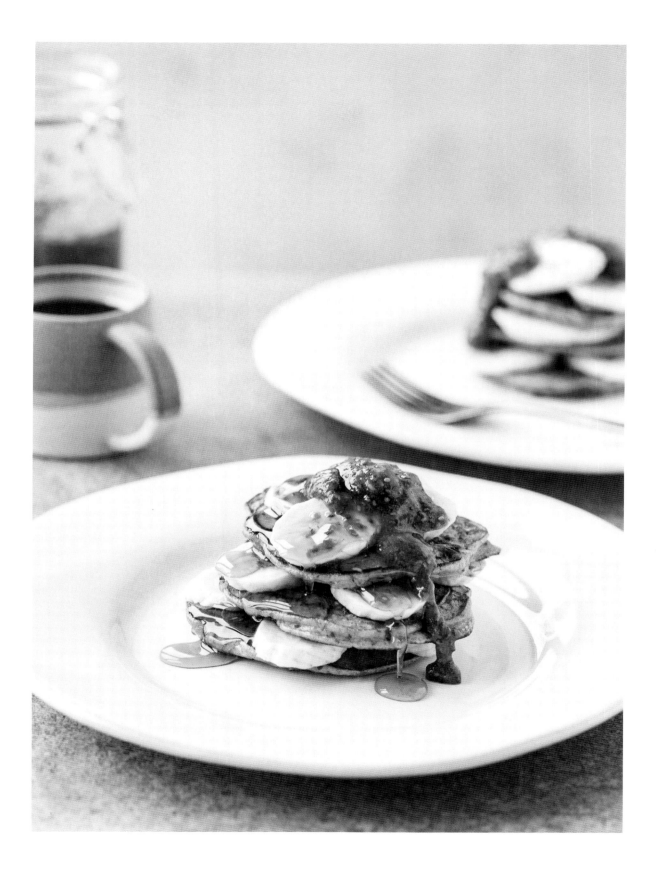

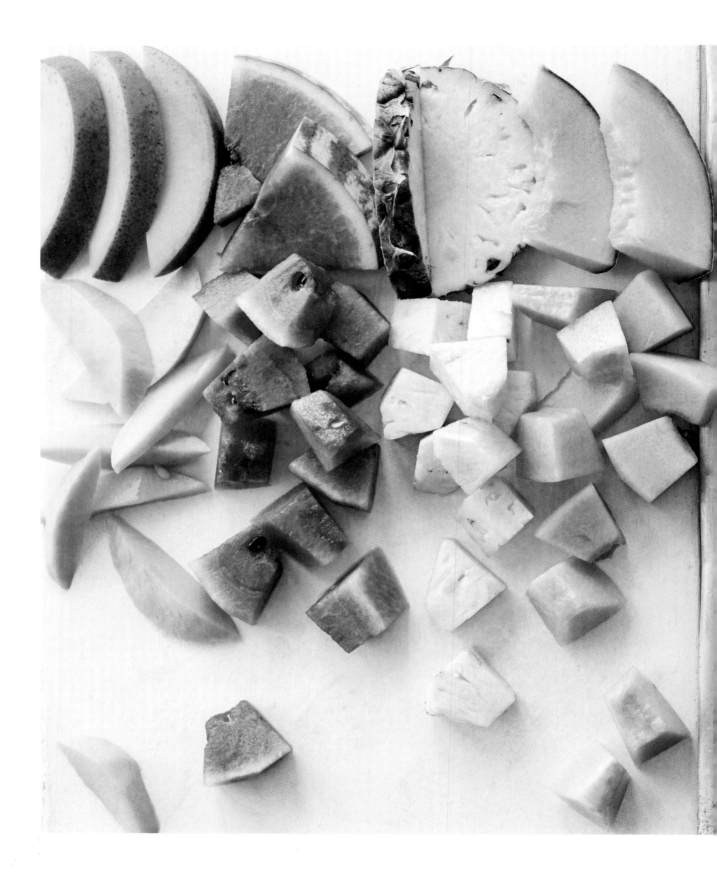

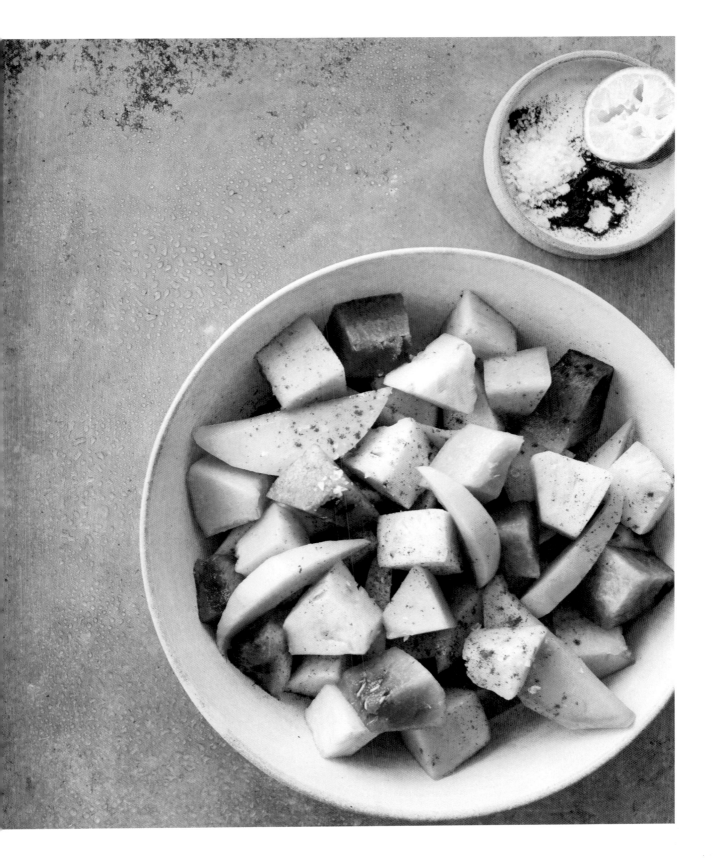

MEXICAN FRUIT SALAD

SERVES 8

In LA, almost every street corner has a pushcart vendor selling some kind of food. One of the most popular things they sell is this really refreshing fruit salad. It may sound strange to add salt and chilli to fruit, but it's really tasty and oddly addictive. Plus, a pinch of chilli powder in the morning is a great way to kick-start the day and I love it before or after a morning run.

1 small, ripe watermelon
1 ripe canteloupe melon
1 ripe mango
1 ripe pineapple
Juice of 1 lime
½–1 tsp chilli powder (optional)
Fine sea salt

1. Prepare all the fruit, removing the skin and pips/stone, and cut the flesh of each into similar bite-sized pieces. Place in a large mixing bowl.

2. Squeeze the lime juice over the fruit pieces and mix well. Add a couple of pinches of salt and mix again so that everything is coated in a little citrus and salt.

3. Transfer to serving bowls, sprinkle each bowl with a little chilli powder, if using, and serve immediately.

PER SERVING	
KCAL	276
FAT (g)	1.0
SATURATES (g)	0.1
CARBS (g)	58.0
SUGARS (g)	53.0
FIBRE (g)	6.0
PROTEIN (g)	5.0
SALT (g)	0.12

GOOD TO KNOW
Watermelon is called watermelon for a reason – it's 92% water! Starting the day with fruit is such a good way to make sure your hydration levels are topped up before you get going.

BAKED ENGLISH BREAKFAST

SERVES 2

A full English breakfast is usually a bit too high in fat to be a good idea after a workout, because fat can slow down the uptake of the vital protein you need for muscle repair after exertion. This tray-baked version, however, is high in protein and lower in fat than a classic fry-up. It's also really easy to put together quickly, which is perfect for when you're in a hurry to refill the empty tank. A bacon medallion is the 'eye' of a rasher of back bacon, so it's the meaty part with the rind and fat removed. If you can't buy them, trim them yourself and use the trimmings for something else.

4 Portobello mushrooms, brushed clean
3 medium tomatoes, halved
1 red onion, peeled and cut in to 8 wedges
4 thyme sprigs, leaves only
2 tbsp olive oil
6 smoked bacon medallions
200g baby spinach
4 eggs
Sea salt and freshly ground black pepper
2 thick slices of toast, to serve

1. Preheat the oven to 200°C/gas 6.

2. Put the mushrooms, gill side up, and the tomatoes, cut side up, on a low-sided roasting tray. Scatter over the onion slices and thyme leaves, then drizzle with the olive oil and sprinkle with salt and pepper.

3. Place the tray in the preheated oven for 20 minutes.

4. After 20 minutes, remove the tray from the oven and pour off any liquid that has been released by the mushrooms. Lay the bacon medallions on top of the other ingredients, then return the tray to the oven to cook for 5 minutes.

5. Meanwhile, bring a kettle of water to boil and put the spinach into a colander over your sink. When boiled, pour the water over the spinach to wilt it. When wilted, run it under cold water, then pick up the leaves in your hands and squeeze out as much excess liquid as you can.

6. Remove the tray from the oven and arrange the spinach leaves on top and around the other ingredients. Make four wells between the spinach and other ingredients and crack the eggs into them.

7. Put the tray back into the oven for another 8 minutes, then remove and serve the baked breakfast with thick slices of toast.

PER SERVING	
KCAL	459
FAT (g)	25.0
SATURATES (g)	5.0
CARBS (g)	14.0
SUGARS (g)	12.0
FIBRE (g)	9.0
PROTEIN (g)	41.0
SALT (g)	0.57

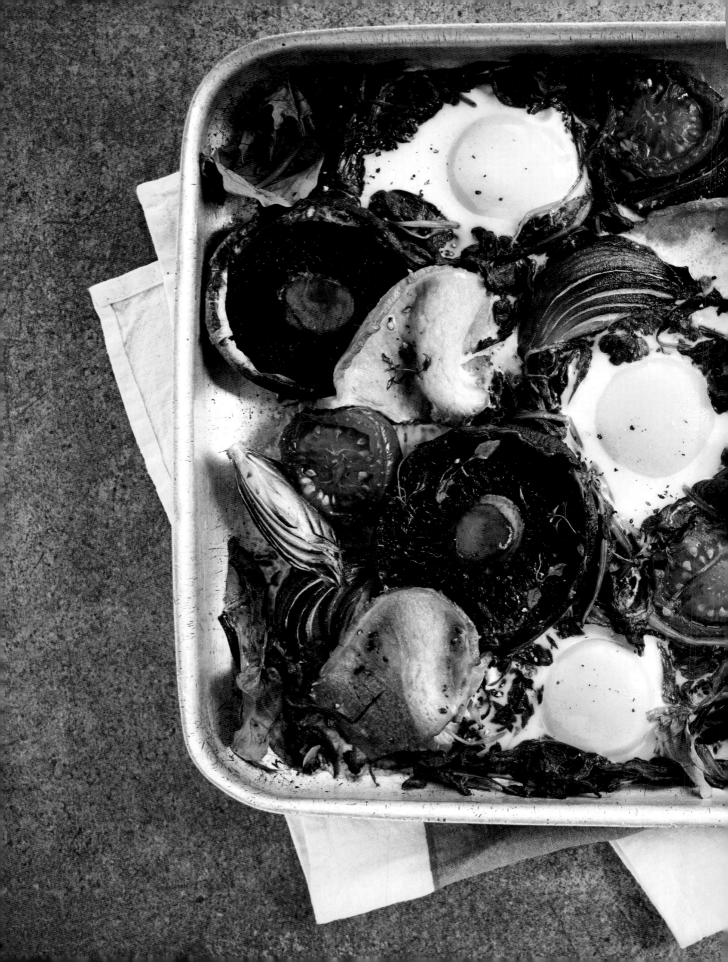

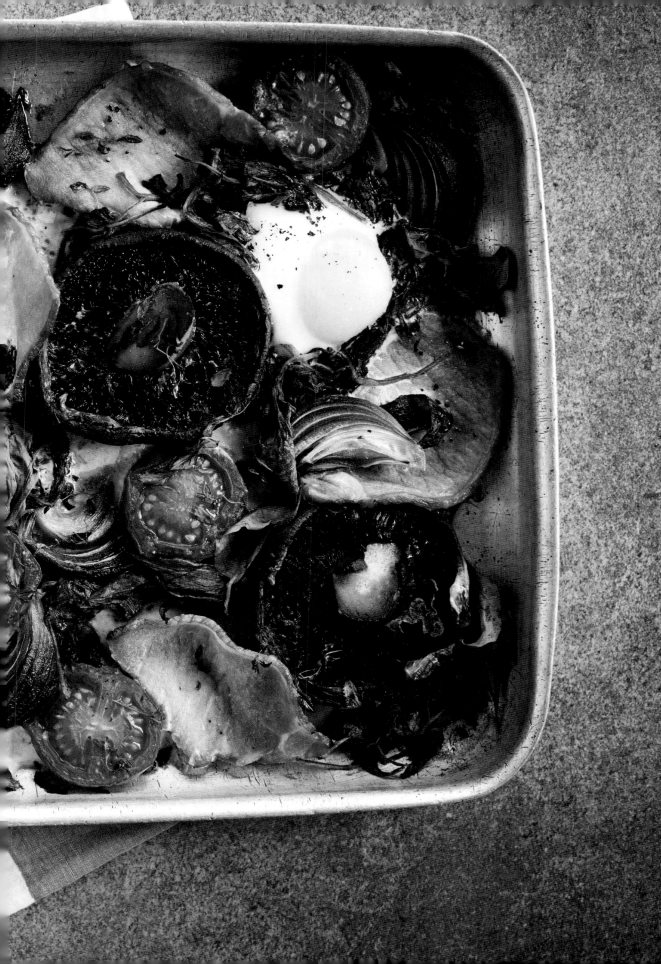

BREAKFAST BURRITO

SERVES 4

A wrap is the ideal portable breakfast if you have an early start. Make these burritos the night before and wrap them in foil to take with you, or enjoy them for brunch after a morning workout. They're packed with strong flavours, lean protein and slow-releasing carbs to meet all your body's nutritional needs pre- or post-exertion.

Olive oil, for frying
½ small red onion (use the remaining half below), diced
1 tsp ground cumin
1 x 400g tin black beans, aduki beans or pinto beans, drained
6 eggs
1 tsp chipotle paste (optional)
4 large seeded wraps
1 ripe avocado, peeled, stoned and sliced
Sea salt and freshly ground black pepper
Mexican hot sauce such as Cholula (optional), to serve

FOR THE SALSA
200g tomatoes, diced
½ small red onion, finely diced (see above)
Juice of ½ lime
Small bunch of coriander, leaves and stalks finely chopped
Dried chilli flakes, to taste

PER SERVING	
KCAL	432
FAT (g)	20.0
SATURATES (g)	5.0
CARBS (g)	38.0
SUGARS (g)	4.0
FIBRE (g)	9.0
PROTEIN (g)	21.0
SALT (g)	1.30

1. Start by making the salsa. Mix all the ingredients together and season with salt and pepper. Taste and add a little more chilli flakes or salt if needed. Put to one side.

2. Place a large frying pan over a medium heat. Add a glug of oil and, once hot, add the diced onion with a pinch of salt. Sweat until translucent and soft, then add the cumin and continue to cook for 1–2 minutes, until fragrant.

3. Add the beans and stir until heated through.

4. Put the eggs into a bowl with the chipotle paste, if using, and beat together with a fork or a whisk until well mixed. Season with a little black pepper. In a second pan, over a medium–low heat, scramble the eggs, stirring now and again until just beginning to set, then remove the pan from the heat and stir them into the beans.

5. Meanwhile, lay the wraps on four plates. Spoon the bean mixture in a horizontal line across the middle of each of the wraps and add a spoonful of salsa. Top with slices of avocado.

6. Fold the sides of each wrap inwards, then roll from the bottom to the top until you have a log, wrapping the filling tightly inside.

7. Serve with a little hot sauce on the side, if desired.

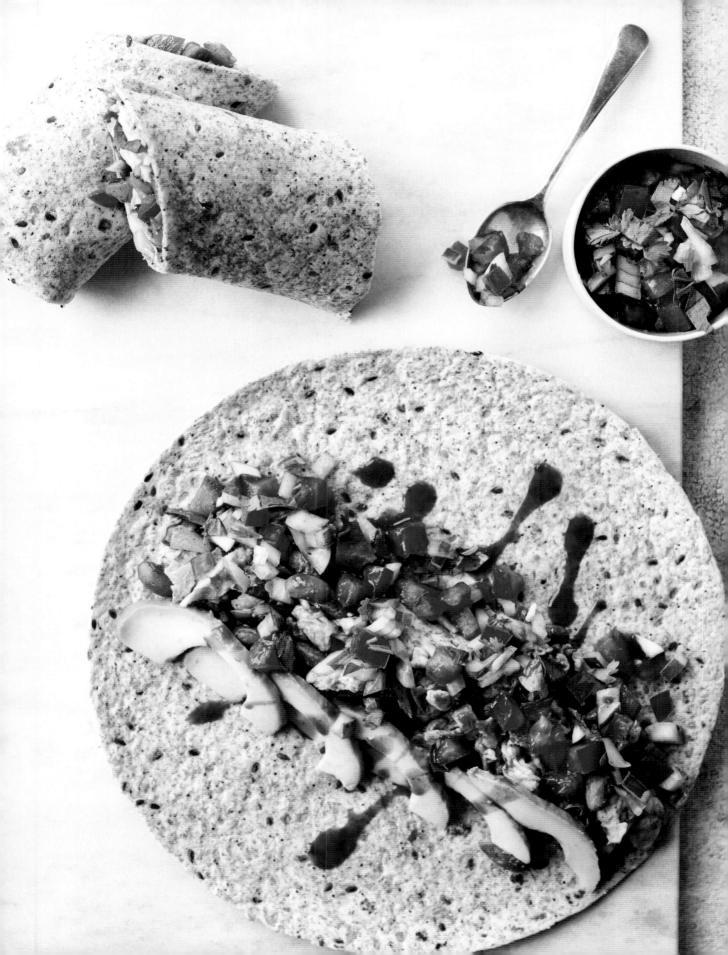

HUEVOS RANCHEROS

SERVES 2

Huevos rancheros is a Mexican breakfast that makes a really substantial brunch before or after a big run or workout. It is really easy to make and excellent for sharing with friends or family. If you don't like too much spice in the morning, leave the chipotle and red chillies out. Personally, I like the kick they give me.

2 x 400g tins chopped tomatoes
20ml olive oil
1 red onion, peeled and diced
1 garlic clove, peeled and sliced
1 green pepper, deseeded and finely diced
1 dried chipotle chilli
1 red chilli, deseeded and finely sliced
4 eggs
2 tortillas, to serve
Small bunch of coriander, roughly chopped
Sea salt and freshly ground black pepper

1. Open one of the tins of tomatoes and tip the contents into a sieve to drain off approximately half the liquid. Set to one side and use the juice for another dish (or in a bloody Mary!).

2. Place a medium frying pan over a medium–high heat and add the oil. When hot, add the red onion, garlic, green pepper and the chipotle and red chillies. Fry the vegetables together for 3 minutes, until just starting to soften.

3. Pour in the drained tomatoes as well as the complete tin of tomatoes, season with salt and pepper, and bring to the boil. Reduce the heat to a simmer and cook for 2 minutes.

4. Make 4 wells in the tomato sauce and crack an egg into each one. Cover with a lid and cook for 8 minutes, until the whites have set but the yolks are still runny.

5. Heat the tortillas according to the packet instructions.

6. Serve the eggs and tomato sauce on top of the warm tortillas with a generous sprinkling of chopped coriander.

PER SERVING	
KCAL	379
FAT (g)	21.0
SATURATES (g)	4.0
CARBS (g)	23.0
SUGARS (g)	21.0
FIBRE (g)	7.0
PROTEIN (g)	21.0
SALT (g)	0.52

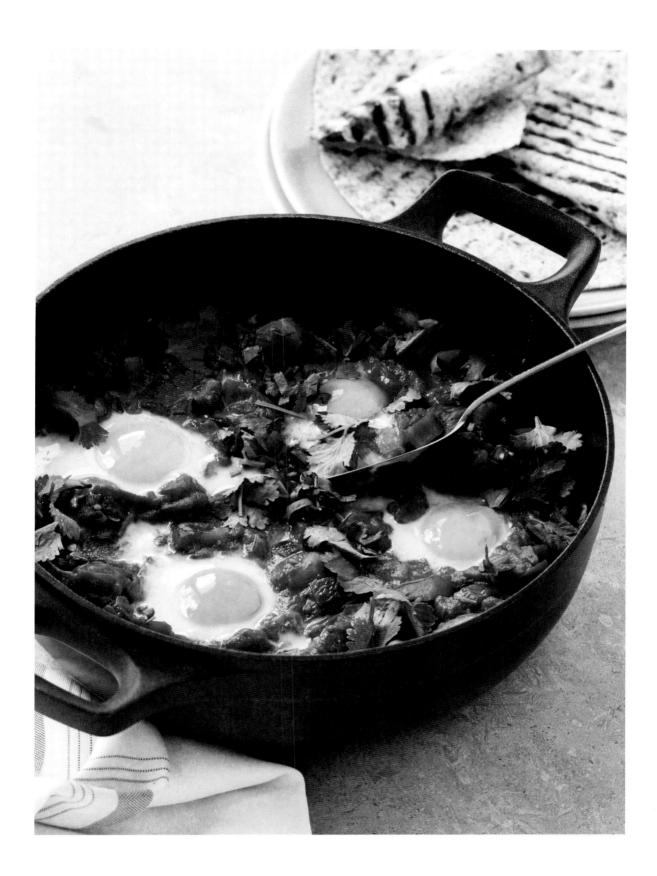

LUNCHES FOR ACTIVE DAYS

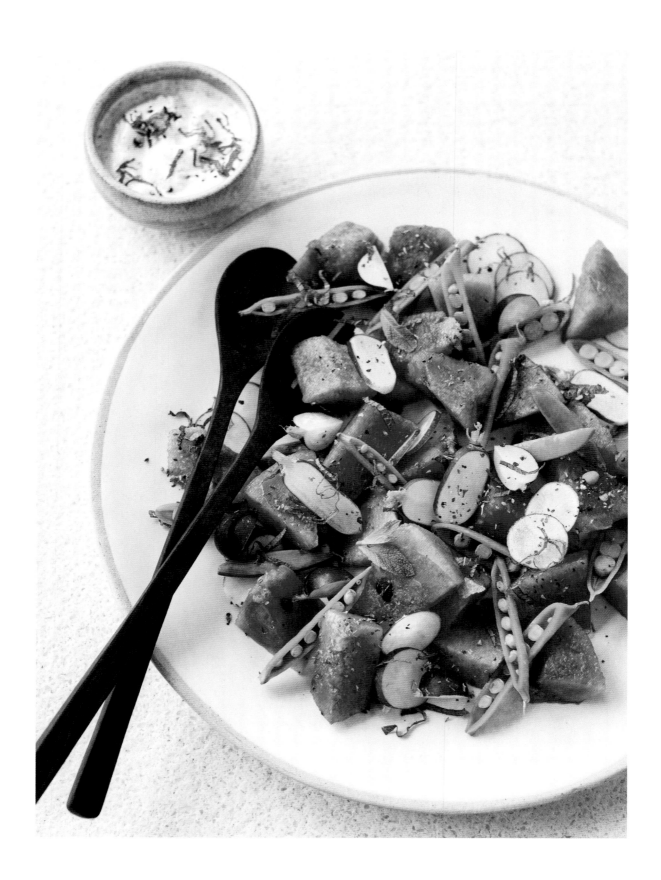

WATERMELON, FETA AND MINT SALAD

SERVES 4

Just because this salad sounds light and healthy doesn't mean it isn't packed with vital energy for active days. The naturally occurring sugars in the fruit, veg and yoghurt are easily accessed by the body but don't overload the system like more difficult-to-digest carbs. Don't make this too far in advance, as the salty cheese will draw the moisture out of the melon and it will lose its crispness.

½ medium watermelon, flesh cut into chunks
100g radishes, trimmed and sliced
100g sugar snap peas or mangetout,
    trimmed and sliced
½ tsp dried oregano
½ small bunch of mint, leaves roughly shredded
Sea salt and freshly ground black pepper

FOR THE DRESSING
75g feta cheese, drained and crumbled
125g natural yoghurt
Dash of water or milk
½ small bunch of mint, leaves finely shredded

1. To make the dressing, put the ingredients into a jug or bowl and blend with a stick blender until smooth. Alternatively, put the feta into a bowl and mash with a fork.

2. Add the yoghurt and mix well, add a dash of water or milk if needed, then stir in the mint leaves. Taste and season with a little pepper.

3. Arrange the watermelon, radishes and sugar snap peas on a serving platter. Sprinkle over the dried oregano and the shredded mint leaves, then drizzle over the feta dressing before serving.

FOR EXTRA PROTEIN
If you want to add some extra protein to this dish, a grilled tuna steak or some squid would be delicious, as would some cooked, peeled king prawns, grilled chicken or lamb kebabs.

PER SERVING	
KCAL	275
FAT (g)	6.0
SATURATES (g)	3.0
CARBS (g)	45.0
SUGARS (g)	39.0
FIBRE (g)	3.0
PROTEIN (g)	9.0
SALT (g)	0.56

WAFER VEGETABLE, CANDIED PECAN AND BLUE CHEESE SALAD

SERVES 4

This crunchy salad is stunning to look at as well as to eat, especially if you manage to get hold of different coloured heirloom beetroots. Choose a firmer blue cheese that crumbles easily, like Stilton, Roquefort or Shropshire Blue, rather than a creamy dolcelatte or Auvergne. Serve with oat cakes or wholemeal or pumpernickel bread for added carbohydrates.

3 raw beetroots, ideally different colours,
    e.g. golden, purple and striped,
    cleaned and peeled
1 green apple
Juice of 1 lemon
75g mooli or radishes
1 head of chicory
2 carrots
3 celery sticks, any leaves reserved
75g blue cheese, crumbled
Sea salt and freshly ground black pepper

FOR THE WALNUT DRESSING
2 tbsp walnut oil
2 tbsp extra virgin olive oil
Juice of 1 lemon
Small bunch of chives, very finely chopped

FOR THE CANDIED PECANS
75g pecans
1 tbsp maple syrup
Pinch of salt

PER SERVING	
KCAL	377
FAT (g)	31.0
SATURATES (g)	6.0
CARBS (g)	15.0
SUGARS (g)	13.0
FIBRE (g)	6.0
PROTEIN (g)	8.0
SALT (g)	0.71

1. Preheat the oven to 170°C/gas 3.

2. First make the candied pecans. Toss the pecans in the maple syrup and season with a pinch of salt. Spread them in a single layer on a baking tray and roast in the preheated oven for 5–7 minutes, turning halfway through, until lightly toasted and caramelized. Watch the nuts carefully so they don't burn. Remove and leave to cool.

3. Meanwhile, prepare the vegetables. The best instrument for this recipe is a mandolin, but use a very sharp knife if you don't have one. Slice the beetroot into wafer-thin rounds and place in a large mixing bowl of cold water (if you are using purple beetroot, put them into a separate bowl to avoid staining).

4. Core the apple, then slice it into wafer-thin rounds and put them into the mixing bowl, adding the lemon juice to prevent it going brown.

5. Slice the mooli and chicory and add to the bowl.

6. Using a vegetable peeler, peel the carrots into long thin ribbons and put them into the bowl with the other vegetables.

7. Slice the celery very finely on the diagonal.

8. Next, make the dressing; whisk together the ingredients with a good pinch of salt and pepper.

9. When ready to serve, drain the vegetables and pat them dry with a clean tea towel or kitchen paper. Put them all into a dry mixing bowl, pour in the dressing and toss gently to coat. Taste and add more seasoning as necessary.

10. Add the crumbled blue cheese and candied pecans and toss again to mix. Transfer to a serving dish and garnish with any reserved celery leaves before serving.

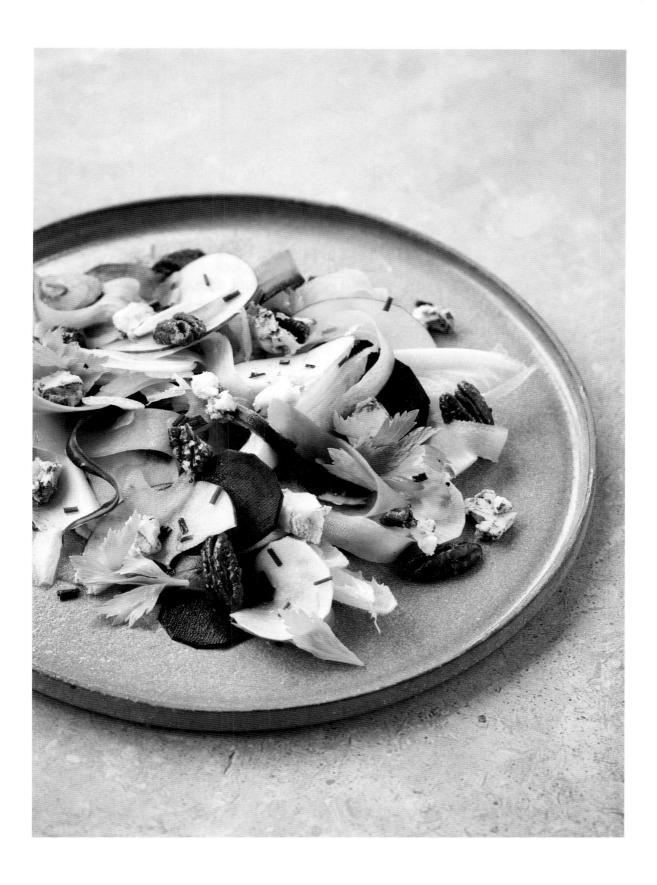

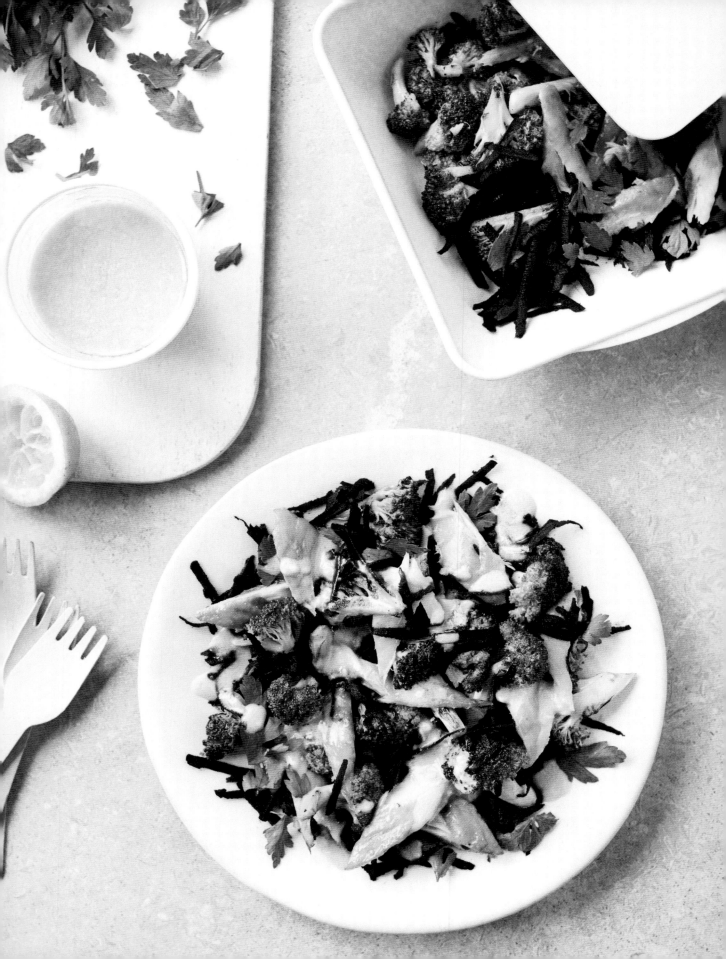

SMOKED MACKEREL, BEETROOT AND BROCCOLI SALAD

SERVES 4

Beetroot is the gym-goer's secret weapon – studies show that eating it and drinking its juice helps you stay the course that little bit longer. Serving them raw is surprisingly delicious and it guarantees that none of the nutrients have been lost through cooking. You could keep the broccoli florets raw, too, but charring them does add a delicious caramelized flavour to the salad. This is a good protein-packed lunch to take with you for post-exercise replenishment.

1 medium head of broccoli, cut into florets
Olive oil, for frying
400g raw beetroot, peeled and grated
4 smoked mackerel fillets
½ small bunch of parsley, leaves roughly chopped
Sea salt and freshly ground black pepper

FOR THE DRESSING
1 tbsp creamed horseradish
Juice of ½ lemon
2 tbsp extra virgin olive oil

1. Heat a large frying pan over a medium heat and add the broccoli florets. Drizzle with a little olive oil and season with salt and pepper. Toss to evenly coat the broccoli with oil. Leave the broccoli in the pan without stirring for 3–4 minutes, until lightly browned on one side. Turn and repeat on the other side. Once charred but still crunchy, remove from the heat.

2. Meanwhile, whisk together the ingredients for the dressing in a small bowl until combined. Taste and adjust the seasoning as necessary, adding more lemon juice if required.

3. Put the grated beetroot on to a serving platter, scatter over the broccoli and gently mix together. Flake over the smoked mackerel fillets, keeping an eye out for bones, then sprinkle with the chopped parsley and gently toss.

4. Drizzle with the dressing and serve immediately, or store covered in the fridge for up to 3 days.

FOR EXTRA ENERGY
Add a handful of cooked lentils, couscous or grains per person if you're carb-loading.

PER SERVING	
KCAL	611
FAT (g)	44.0
SATURATES (g)	8.0
CARBS (g)	12.0
SUGARS (g)	10.0
FIBRE (g)	8.0
PROTEIN (g)	39.0
SALT (g)	3.08

SUSHI SALAD BOWL

SERVES 4

This is a great way to get all the flavours of sushi without any of the hassle of making it. The seaweed isn't essential, but given that it provides an impressive amount of valuable nutrients as well as a mouth-pleasing umami hit, it is definitely worth experimenting with. Although this is very filling as it is, you can up the protein content by adding smoked or raw salmon, tuna, prawns or other flaked fish.

1 head of broccoli, cut into small florets
2 tbsp dried seaweed such as dulse or
    wakame (if unavailable, replace with
    3 crumbled sheets of nori)
400g cooked and cooled brown rice
    (approx. 100g–125g uncooked rice)
1 cucumber, deseeded and sliced
2 ripe avocados, peeled, stoned and sliced
50g sushi ginger, cut into strips
2 tbsp sesame seeds, black or white
Small bunch of chives, finely chopped
2 tbsp soy sauce
4 tsp brown rice vinegar
2 tsp toasted sesame oil

1. Blanch the broccoli florets by plunging them into boiling salted water for 2 minutes until the rawness has been removed but they are still crunchy. Refresh immediately in cold water to prevent further cooking. Chop into bite-sized pieces once cooked.

2. Meanwhile soak the dried seaweed in a bowl of warm water for 5 minutes or until soft (if using crumbled nori, you do not need to soak them). Drain once soft.

3. Divide the rice between four serving bowls, pushing it to one side so it takes up a quarter of the bowl. Add the cooled broccoli to another quarter. Add the cucumber and avocado in the same way and then the seaweed. (If you're using crumbled nori, sprinkle it over the top with the sesame seeds in step 4.)

4. Sprinkle over the sushi ginger strips, sesame seeds and chopped chives. Drizzle each bowl with a little soy sauce and add a couple of drops of rice vinegar and sesame oil before serving.

PER SERVING	
KCAL	411
FAT (g)	21.0
SATURATES (g)	4.0
CARBS (g)	36.0
SUGARS (g)	5.0
FIBRE (g)	12.0
PROTEIN (g)	14.0
SALT (g)	1.39

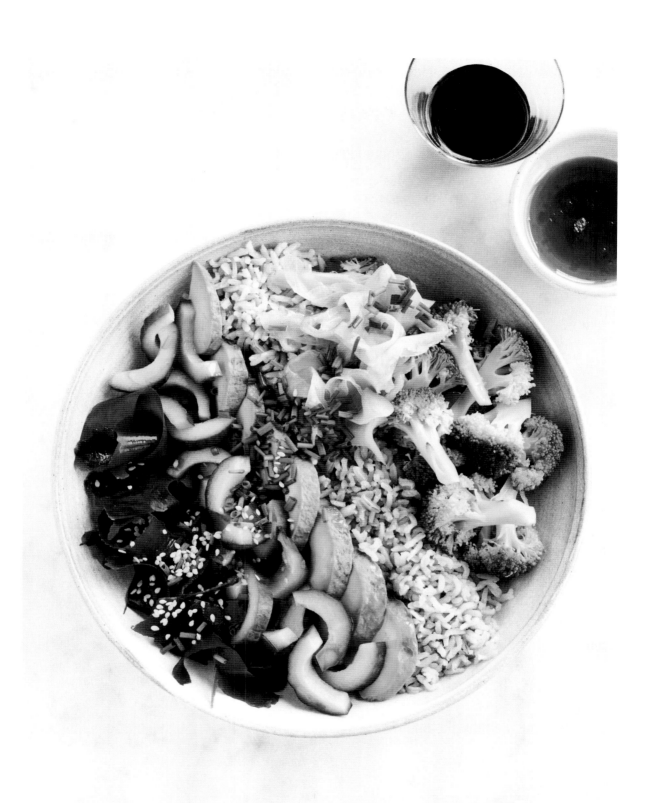

VIETNAMESE CRISPY TOFU WRAP

SERVES 4

The flavours in this recipe are taken from the popular Vietnamese sandwich, bánh mì, but I've ditched the meat in favour of baked, marinated tofu and replaced the white baguette with a wholemeal wrap. Same great taste but better energy sources for exercise. The pickled vegetables and the sriracha yoghurt dressing are both great things to have on standby in your fridge to perk up almost any meal.

350g firm tofu, drained
1 tbsp fish sauce
Juice of ½ lime
2 tsp agave syrup
4 tbsp natural yoghurt
1 tsp sriracha chilli sauce
4 large wholemeal tortilla wraps
1 baby gem lettuce, shredded
½ cucumber, julienned
Small bunch of coriander, leaves roughly torn

FOR THE PICKLED VEGETABLES
125ml rice wine vinegar
2 tsp agave syrup
1 carrot, peeled and julienned
½ daikon radish, julienned (if unavailable, use 6 radishes, trimmed and sliced)

PER SERVING	
KCAL	322
FAT (g)	10.0
SATURATES (g)	3.0
CARBS (g)	37.0
SUGARS (g)	11.0
FIBRE (g)	7.0
PROTEIN (g)	17.0
SALT (g)	1.88

VARIATIONS
You can change the flavour of the tofu by altering the marinade: try a little miso paste let down with a dash of soy sauce and rice vinegar or a mixture of soy and hoisin sauce. And if you really don't like tofu, you can swap it for marinated chicken pieces or prawns.

1. For the pickled vegetables, mix together the rice wine vinegar and agave syrup in a wide, shallow bowl, then stir in the carrots and radishes and cover. Leave to pickle for a minimum of 30 minutes and up to 48 hours.

2. Preheat the oven to 170°C/gas 3.

3. Put the tofu on a plate between two layers of kitchen paper and place a heavy object such as a cast-iron pan on top. Press for 20 minutes to remove excess liquid.

4. Once the tofu has been pressed, slice it into bite-sized pieces.

5. Mix together the fish sauce, lime juice and agave syrup and toss the tofu pieces in the marinade until each piece is coated.

6. Place the tofu in a single layer on a non-stick baking tray and bake in the preheated oven for 20–25 minutes, turning occasionally until crisp and golden on all sides but still soft in the middle.

7. Meanwhile, mix together the yoghurt and sriracha sauce until combined.

8. Once the tofu is cooked, remove the tray from the oven. Spread a little of the sriracha yoghurt on to each tortilla wrap, then scatter over some baby gem lettuce, cucumber matchsticks and coriander leaves. Top with the baked tofu and add some pickled vegetables, drizzling with a little of the pickling liquor.

9. Add a dollop of extra sriracha yoghurt, then fold the sides of the tortilla inwards and roll from the bottom to the top until you have a log, wrapping the filling tightly inside. Slice in half on the diagonal to serve.

CALIFORNIAN 'FRIED' CHICKEN SANDWICH

SERVES 4

As a family with four teenage children, we are always looking for healthy ways of preparing not-so-healthy fast food favourites like pizza, burgers and fried chicken. This recipe is brilliant because it looks and tastes like a fried chicken sandwich, with the satisfying crunch from the chicken and the creaminess of the mayo, but is actually made with baked chicken and a yoghurt dressing. The kids love it, we know they're eating well and everyone's happy.

50g wholemeal flour
200ml buttermilk (or 2 eggs, beaten)
150g puffed rice
2 tsp garlic powder
2 tsp onion powder or granules
4 tsp paprika
1 tsp dried sage
8 mini chicken breast fillets
4 wholemeal buns
1 ripe avocado, peeled, stoned and sliced
½ iceberg lettuce, shredded
Sea salt and freshly ground black pepper
Mexican hot sauce such as Cholula (optional), to serve

FOR THE YOGHURT DRESSING
75ml Greek yoghurt
½ garlic clove, crushed
1 tsp cider vinegar

1. Preheat the oven to 180°C/gas 4.

2. Put the flour, buttermilk and puffed rice into three shallow bowls. Season the flour with salt and pepper. Add the garlic powder, onion powder, paprika and dried sage to the buttermilk and mix well. Crush the puffed rice with your hands so that the pieces are broken down slightly but not powdered.

3. Dip a piece of chicken into the flour so that it is completely covered. Remove and shake off any excess, then dip into the buttermilk. Allow any excess buttermilk to drip off, then put the chicken pieces into the puffed rice. Turn over to make sure they are completely coated, then place on a baking tray. Repeat with the remaining chicken pieces.

4. Put the tray into the preheated oven and bake for 25–30 minutes, until golden and cooked through, turning halfway through cooking.

5. Meanwhile, make the yoghurt dressing; mix together the yoghurt, crushed garlic and vinegar with a little salt and pepper. Taste and add more vinegar if needed.

6. Slice open the buns and divide the avocado slices between them. Top with shredded iceberg lettuce.

7. Once the chicken is cooked, place on top of the lettuce and spoon over dollops of the yoghurt dressing, as well as a drizzle of hot sauce, if desired. Close the buns and serve immediately.

PER SERVING	
KCAL	510
FAT (g)	13.0
SATURATES (g)	4.0
CARBS (g)	67.0
SUGARS (g)	10.0
FIBRE (g)	8.0
PROTEIN (g)	27.0
SALT (g)	1.30

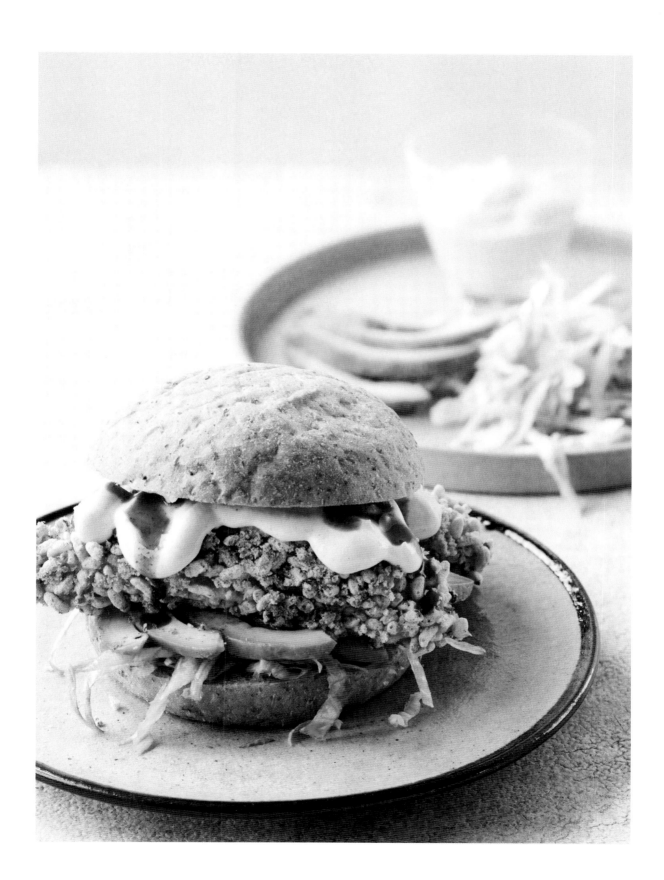

CARB-LOADING FOR THE NIGHT BEFORE

SAKE-AND-MISO-STEAMED MUSSELS WITH SOBA NOODLES

SERVES 4

This is a Japanese take on the French classic moules marinières but without all the cream. Soba noodles are made from buckwheat flour, which is naturally fat- and gluten-free and provides lots of starchy carbohydrate for filling up the tank before a challenge. The noodles soak up all the delicious juices brilliantly, but miso is quite salty so make sure you drink plenty of water at the same time. Also, the remains of the bottle of sake would be delicious served with this dish if you aren't running a marathon the following day!

2kg fresh mussels
200g soba noodles
125g tenderstem broccoli
1 tbsp flavourless oil, e.g. groundnut
1 banana shallot, peeled and finely sliced
2cm piece of fresh root ginger,
   peeled and grated
2 garlic cloves, peeled and sliced
1 tbsp miso paste
250ml sake

1. To test that the mussels are OK to eat, place them in a sink or a large bowl of cold water. Throw away any that do not close when tapped against a hard surface. Drain the mussels and remove the beards.

2. Fill a medium saucepan with hot water and bring to the boil. Add the soba noodles and cook for 4 minutes, then add the tenderstem broccoli. After 2–3 minutes taste the soba noodles and, if done (tender with no bite but not soggy), drain in a colander and divide between four serving bowls with the cooked broccoli.

3. Meanwhile, to cook the mussels, place a large heavy-based casserole dish or saucepan with a tight-fitting lid over a medium heat. Add the oil and, once hot, fry the shallot, ginger and garlic for 2 minutes, until the shallot begins to soften.

4. Add the miso paste and stir. Increase the heat, then add the sake and stir into the paste. Bubble for 2 minutes to burn off the alcohol, then tip in the mussels. Stir the mussels to coat them in the liquid, then put the lid on and cook for 3–4 minutes, shaking the pan occasionally until all the mussels are open. Discard any that have not opened after cooking.

5. Divide the mussels and the cooking liquor between the four bowls of noodles and serve immediately.

PER SERVING	
KCAL	439
FAT (g)	7.0
SATURATES (g)	1.0
CARBS (g)	43.0
SUGARS (g)	1.0
FIBRE (g)	1.0
PROTEIN (g)	34.0
SALT (g)	2.75

GOOD TO KNOW
Mussels are a valuable source of energizing iron – in fact, they contain more iron per 100g than red meat!

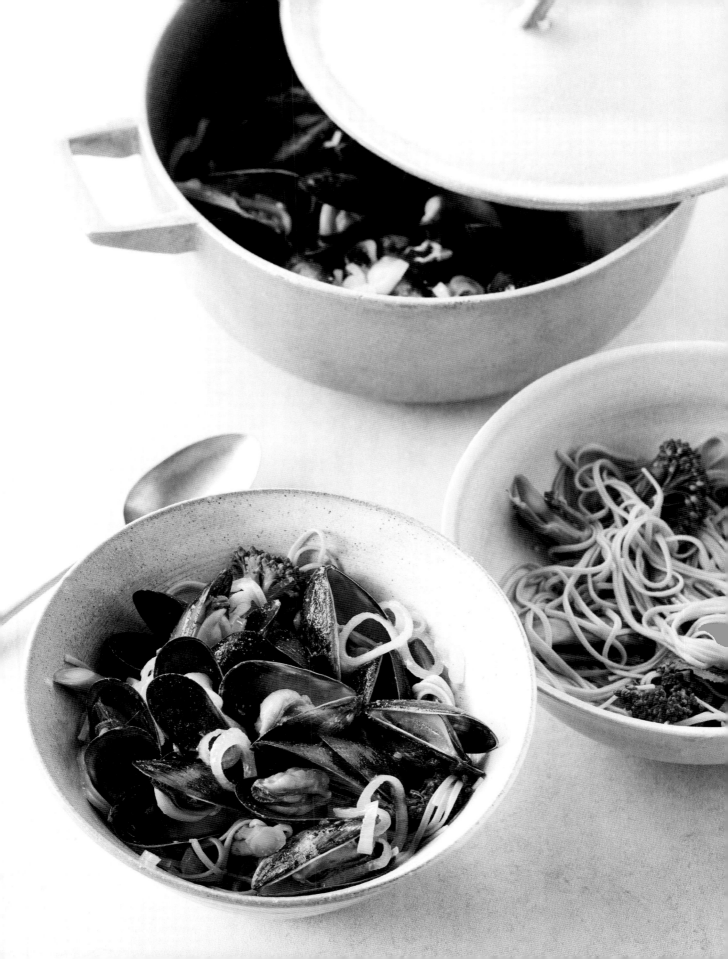

SOUTHERN INDIAN FISH CURRY

SERVES 6

This is a lightly spiced, creamy curry with a delicately sweet-and-sour flavour that is popular in the southern regions of India. Serve it with boiled basmati or brown rice for a perfectly balanced pre-exercise meal. Coconut is rich in a certain type of saturated fat which is metabolized more rapidly than that from animal sources – this means that coconut makes a useful energy source for endurance sport and competitions.

½ tbsp flavourless oil, e.g. groundnut, for frying
2 onions, peeled and finely sliced
2 tsp mustard seeds
1 tsp ground turmeric
2 tsp ground cumin
3cm piece of fresh root ginger, peeled and grated
1–2 long red chillies, deseeded and finely chopped, to taste
1 x 400ml tin reduced fat coconut milk
1–2 tbsp tamarind paste or watered-down tamarind block (see tip on page 151)
1 small aubergine, cut into bite-sized pieces
2 carrots, chopped into bite-sized rounds
200g green beans, topped and tailed and cut in half
600g meaty white fish (e.g. cod, pollock, haddock or coley), cut into bite-sized pieces
Sea salt and freshly ground black pepper

TO SERVE
Coconut and Ginger Brown Rice (see opposite)
2 tbsp desiccated coconut, toasted (optional)

KCAL	342
FAT (g)	8.0
SATURATES (g)	5.0
CARBS (g)	42.0
SUGARS (g)	7.0
FIBRE (g)	5.0
PROTEIN (g)	23.0
SALT (g)	0.22

1. Place a large, shallow saucepan or a high-sided frying pan over a medium heat and add the oil. Once hot, add the sliced onions with a pinch of salt and sauté for 8–10 minutes, until completely soft.

2. Add the spices and continue to cook for a further minute or until you can really smell them, then add the ginger and chillies and stir over the heat for a further minute.

3. Pour in the coconut milk, tamarind paste and 400ml of water (use the empty coconut milk tin to measure the 400ml). Season with salt and pepper, stir well and bring to a simmer.

4. Once the sauce is simmering, add the aubergine and continue to cook for 5 minutes, then add the carrots and simmer for 10–15 minutes, until the carrots and aubergine are tender and the sauce has thickened a little.

5. Add the green beans and cook for a further 3 minutes, then add the fish. Stir well to coat, then cook for 3–4 minutes, until the fish is just cooked through. Taste and adjust the seasoning as necessary.

6. Serve the curry with rice in warmed serving bowls, sprinkled with toasted desiccated coconut, if using.

COCONUT AND GINGER BROWN RICE

SERVES 6 AS A SIDE

This rich and fragrant rice is delicious with curries or as a side to any Asian main course, and it makes a great change from plain boiled rice. Cooking the rice in coconut milk does increase the level of fat and saturated fat in the dish, but there are advantages to using coconut that make this an excellent choice for a pre-event supper.

1 tbsp rapeseed oil, for frying
1 small onion, peeled and finely diced
3cm piece of fresh root ginger,
    peeled and grated
1 tsp ground turmeric
300g brown basmati rice
1 x 400ml tin reduced fat coconut milk
Chopped coriander, to serve (optional)
Sea salt

1. Place a medium heavy-based saucepan over a medium heat. Add the rapeseed oil and, once hot, add the finely diced onion with a pinch of salt. Cook for 5–6 minutes, until softened.

2. Add the ginger and turmeric and continue to cook for 2 minutes, stirring everything together. Then stir in the rice, ensuring it is well coated in the flavoured oil.

3. Pour in the coconut milk and 400ml of boiling water and bring up to a simmer. Simmer for 5 minutes, then reduce the heat to low and cover with a lid. Cook for a further 30–35 minutes, until the rice is tender and the liquid has been absorbed.

4. Remove the rice from the heat and fluff with a fork, seasoning with a pinch of salt if needed. Serve immediately, sprinkled with coriander, if using.

HOW TO USE UP LEFTOVER RICE
Leftover rice can be stir-fried the next day with added vegetables, eggs, meat, prawns or tofu for a delicious lunch or supper.

PER SERVING	
KCAL	289
FAT (g)	9.0
SATURATES (g)	5.0
CARBS (g)	45.0
SUGARS (g)	2.0
FIBRE (g)	2.0
PROTEIN (g)	6.0
SALT (g)	0.0

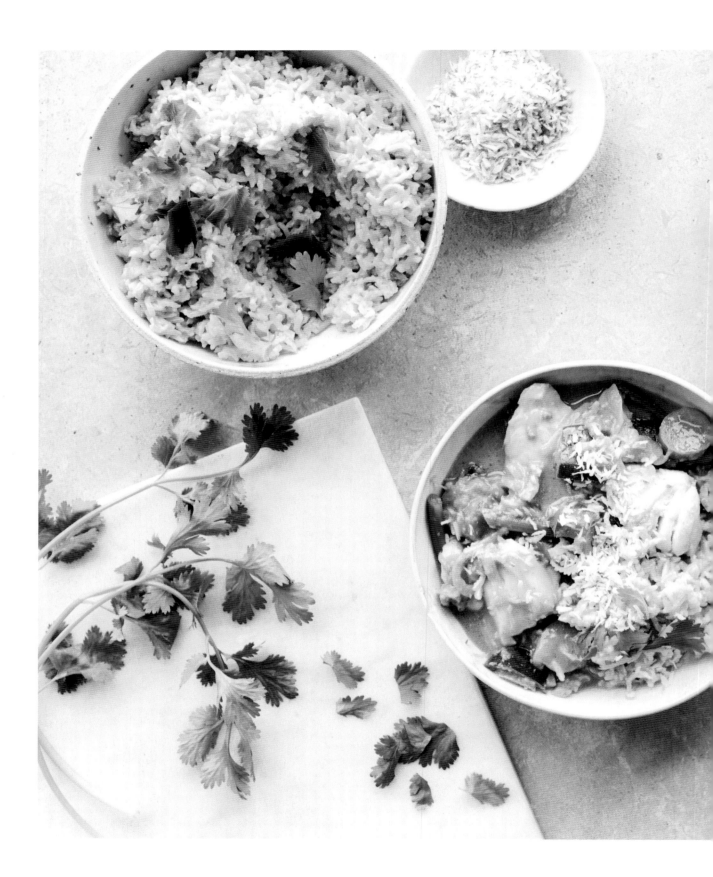

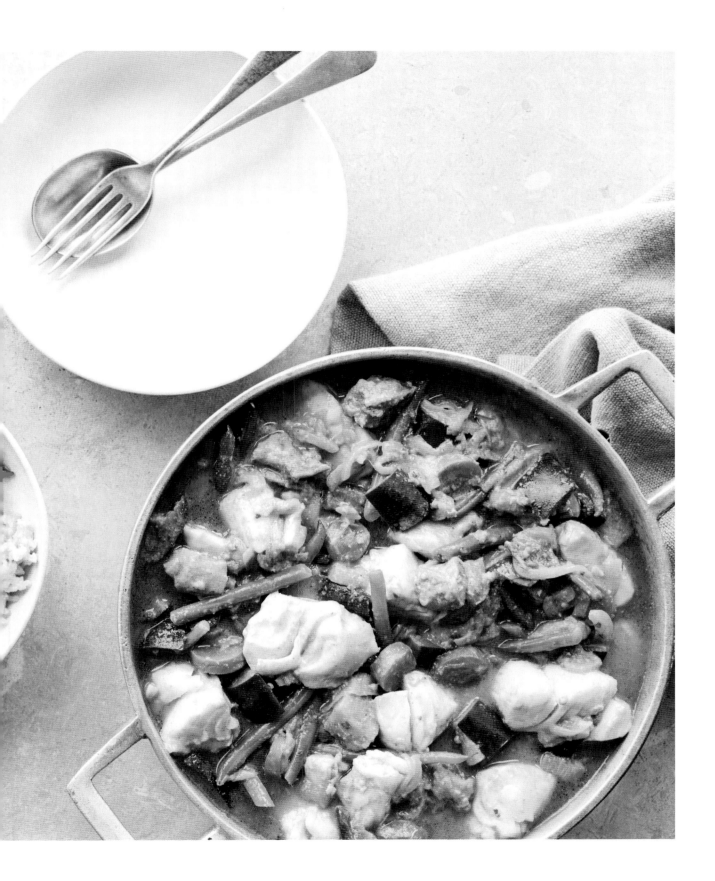

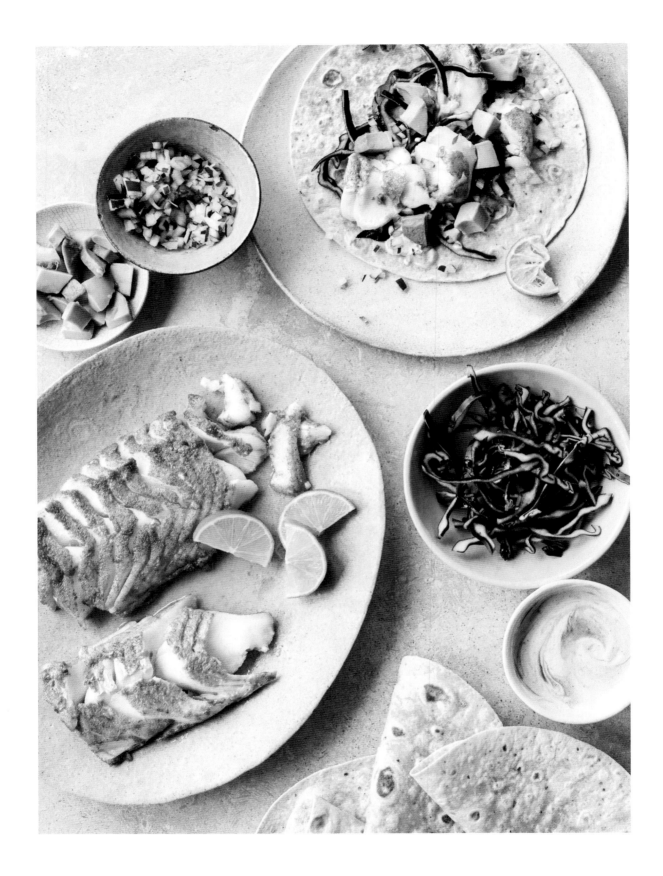

SPICED FISH TACOS

SERVES 4

We love tacos in my house, particularly because everyone has their individual preferences when it comes to Mexican food. My son, Jack, for example, loves things really, really hot, while his twin sister, Holly, likes to keep it much milder. Therefore, we put all the different components on the table and get everyone to help themselves to their own perfect taco. These are brilliant to serve before a race or match day because each individual can eat as many tacos as they need depending on whether they are taking part or not.

100g natural yoghurt
½ tbsp chipotle paste, or to taste
¼ small red cabbage, finely shredded
1 small red onion, peeled and finely diced
1 ripe avocado, peeled, stoned and roughly
   chopped
2 limes, cut into wedges
12 small, soft corn taco tortillas or 4 large ones
2 tsp ground cumin
1 tsp smoked paprika
1½ tbsp rice or plain flour
300g meaty white fish fillets,
   skin removed and pin-boned
Coconut oil or flavourless oil,
   e.g. groundnut, for frying
Sea salt and freshly ground black pepper

1. Mix together the yoghurt and chipotle paste. If you prefer a slightly hotter chipotle sauce, add a little more than half a tablespoon. Put into a small serving bowl and set aside.

2. Put the shredded cabbage, red onion, avocado and lime wedges each in their own bowls and set aside.

3. Place a large frying pan over a medium heat. Have a bowl of water next to the pan and put the tortillas into the pan two at a time for 2 minutes to heat through. As they heat, sprinkle them with a little water by dipping your fingers in the bowl of water and flicking it at the tortillas. Turn the tortillas halfway through, then wrap them in a clean tea towel to stay warm while you heat the rest.

4. Mix together the ground cumin, smoked paprika and flour and season with a pinch of salt and pepper. Dip the fish fillets into the spiced flour, making sure they are well covered.

5. Heat a tablespoon of coconut oil in the frying pan and, once hot, fry the fish for 2–4 minutes on each side (depending on thickness of the fillets), until just cooked through. Remove from the heat.

6. Flake the fish into bite-sized chunks and put them on to a serving plate. Bring to the table with the vegetables, sauce, limes and tortillas and get everyone to build their own tacos.

VARIATIONS

This is a great recipe for trying out new varieties of fish that you might not usually buy. Try whiting, pollock, hake, coley or gurnard to make a change from the usual haddock or cod.

PER SERVING	
KCAL	575
FAT (g)	19.0
SATURATES (g)	5.0
CARBS (g)	73.0
SUGARS (g)	5.0
FIBRE (g)	4.0
PROTEIN (g)	26.0
SALT (g)	2.86

CHICKEN AND CHICKPEA TAGINE

SERVES 4

As well as carbohydrates, my training diet focuses on lean protein like chicken and fish. It's a simple menu that can get quite repetitive, which is why I like rich braises like this tagine. It's deeply tasty, very filling and easy to digest. The chickpeas and couscous are a brilliant source of carbohydrate and the spices stop my taste buds getting bored – it's a win–win.

1.25 litres chicken stock
400g couscous
Pinch of saffron
Olive oil, for frying and drizzling
1kg chicken thighs, skin removed
2 onions, peeled and diced
2 garlic cloves, peeled and finely sliced
1 cinnamon stick
2 tsp ground coriander
1 tsp ground turmeric
2 preserved lemons, finely chopped
2 x 400g tins chickpeas, drained and rinsed
40g pitted black olives, halved
2 spring onions, trimmed and finely sliced
6 radishes, trimmed and quartered
Large bunch of parsley, roughly chopped
Sea salt and freshly ground black pepper

1. Put the chicken stock into a saucepan and bring to the boil.

2. Tip the couscous into a large bowl and pour over 500ml of the boiling chicken stock. Cover the bowl with cling film and leave to stand. Add the saffron to the remaining chicken stock and leave to infuse.

3. Place a large casserole over a medium–high heat and add a little olive oil. When hot, add half the chicken thighs and cook until golden brown all over, then remove them to a plate. Add a little more oil if needed, then repeat the process with the remaining chicken thighs.

4. Reduce the heat under the casserole to medium and add the onions, garlic and cinnamon stick. Sauté for 8–10 minutes, until the onions are very soft and have turned translucent. If you feel that the onions are catching on the base of the pan, add a splash of water to deglaze rather than more oil.

5. Stir in the coriander, turmeric and chopped preserved lemon and continue to sauté for 1 minute, stirring occasionally.

6. Return the browned chicken thighs to the pan, then pour over the infused chicken stock. Bring to the boil, then reduce to a simmer for 20 minutes.

7. After 20 minutes, add the chickpeas and olives to the casserole and continue to cook for a further 15 minutes, until the chicken is cooked through and the chickpeas are soft.

8. Meanwhile, remove the cling film from the top of the couscous and add the chopped spring onions, radishes, a drizzle of olive oil and half the chopped parsley. Season well with salt and pepper.

9. Stir the remaining chopped parsley into the tagine and serve with the couscous.

PER SERVING	
KCAL	902
FAT (g)	27.0
SATURATES (g)	5.0
CARBS (g)	101.0
SUGARS (g)	8.0
FIBRE (g)	16.0
PROTEIN (g)	56.0
SALT (g)	1.09

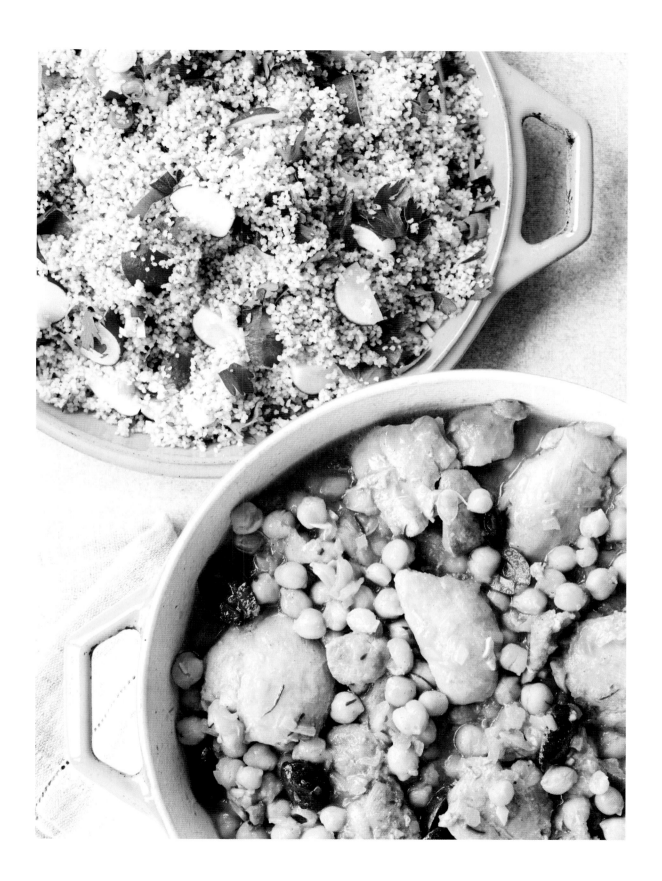

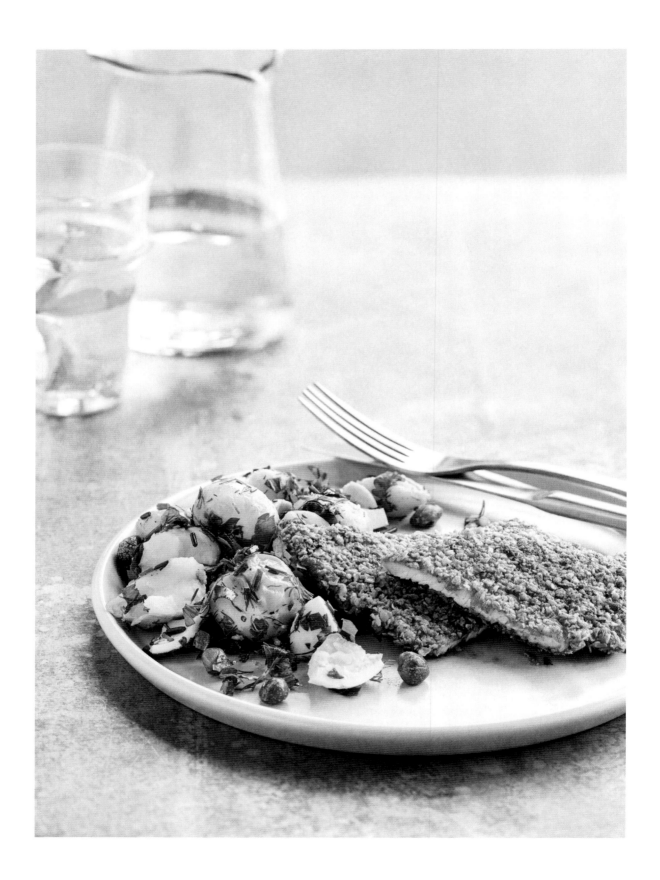

CRISPY SPICED TURKEY WITH EGG AND POTATO SALAD

SERVES 2

Finding ways to load up on carbohydrates without relying on pasta and baked potatoes can be challenging. This crispy turkey is coated with oats and served with a herby new potato salad that will make carb-loading a doddle. When bashing the turkey, keeping its shape isn't as important as getting an even thickness all over so don't worry if it looks a bit strange.

2 turkey breasts, skin removed
125g porridge oats
3 tsp sweet smoked paprika
2 eggs
40g plain flour
300g new potatoes
40ml olive oil
Small bunch of dill, roughly chopped
Small bunch of parsley, roughly chopped
Small bunch of chives, finely chopped
2 tsp capers
Sea salt and freshly ground black pepper
Rocket leaves, to serve

1. Lay a piece of cling film over your chopping board and place a turkey breast on top. Lay a second piece of cling film over the top and, using a meat mallet or rolling pin, bash the breast until it is about 1cm thick all over. Repeat this process with the second breast.

2. Mix the porridge oats with the smoked paprika then scatter them over a large plate.

3. Crack one of the eggs into a shallow bowl and beat with a fork. Pour the flour on to a second plate and season well with salt and pepper.

4. Dip the flattened breasts into the flour one at a time, then dip them into the egg and finally coat them in the spiced porridge oats. Keep the breasts in the fridge while you prepare the potatoes.

CONTINUED OVERLEAF

PER SERVING	
KCAL	859
FAT (g)	32.0
SATURATES (g)	6.0
CARBS (g)	80.0
SUGARS (g)	3.0
FIBRE (g)	12.0
PROTEIN (g)	57.0
SALT (g)	0.62

CONTINUED FROM PAGE 239

5. Bring a pan of water to the boil and simmer the potatoes for 5 minutes then add the second egg and continue to cook for 10 minutes, until the potatoes are cooked through.

6. Drain the egg and potatoes in a colander then immediately run the egg under cold running water to cool it down.

7. When the potatoes are well drained, tip them into a large bowl. When cool enough to handle, peel and finely chop the egg and add it to the potatoes. Give them a rough stir with a fork to break open some of the potatoes, then while still warm, pour in a tablespoon of the olive oil, the chopped dill, parsley, chives and capers along with a good pinch of salt and pepper. Toss everything gently together then leave to one side.

8. Place a large, non-stick frying pan over a medium-high heat and add the remaining olive oil. When it is hot, carefully slide the coated turkey into the pan and cook for 4 minutes on each side or until you are sure they are cooked through.

9. Serve the coated turkey with the salad and a handful of rocket leaves.

SWEET POTATO CHIPS WITH CHERMOULA

SERVES 4 AS A SIDE

As well as being carbohydrate-rich, sweet potatoes have many health benefits that regular potatoes do not – for example, they have more fibre and vitamins A and C than the common spud. Leaving the skin on and baking these chips also makes them better for you than unhealthy French fries. Chermoula is a punchy North African sauce that goes really well with the sweetness of the sweet potatoes, but leave it out if it clashes with the rest of your menu. These are great with the Californian 'Fried' Chicken Sandwich on page 224 or with steak, burgers or sausages.

3 sweet potatoes, scrubbed
1 tbsp olive oil
Sea salt and freshly ground black pepper

FOR THE CHERMOULA
½–1 tsp smoked paprika, to taste
Juice of ½–1 lemon, to taste
Large bunch of coriander
Small bunch of flat-leaf parsley, leaves only
2 garlic cloves, peeled and roughly chopped
2cm piece of fresh root ginger,
    peeled and roughly chopped
½ red chilli, deseeded and roughly chopped
    (optional)
2 tsp ground cumin
Olive oil

1. Preheat the oven to 190°C/gas 5.

2. Cut the sweet potatoes into chips about 1cm wide, leaving the skin on.

3. Put the chips into a large mixing bowl, drizzle over the olive oil and season with salt and pepper. Toss well to make sure that each chip is coated with oil, then spread them in a single layer on two baking trays. Put the trays into the preheated oven and bake for 15 minutes, then remove from the oven and turn the chips over. Return to the oven for a further 7–10 minutes, until all the chips are golden.

4. While the chips are cooking, make the chermoula. Put all the ingredients except the oil into a food processor (starting with ½ tsp of smoked paprika and the juice of ½ lemon) and blend until very finely chopped.

5. With the motor running, pour in enough olive oil (roughly 50ml) to bring the chermoula to a dipping consistency. Taste and adjust the amount of lemon juice and smoked paprika as necessary. Season with salt and pepper and blitz again to mix together.

6. Serve the hot chips with the chermoula dip. Any leftover chermoula can be stored covered in the fridge for up to a week.

HOW TO USE CHERMOULA
You can also use the chermoula to marinate meats and fish – just reduce the amount of oil in this recipe so the result is a stiffer paste.

PER SERVING	
KCAL	318
FAT (g)	16.0
SATURATES (g)	2.0
CARBS (g)	36.0
SUGARS (g)	19.0
FIBRE (g)	3.0
PROTEIN (g)	7.0
SALT (g)	0.19

HIGH-PROTEIN RECOVERY MEALS FOR THE EVENING AFTER

CAULIFLOWER PIZZA

SERVES 2 (MAKES 1 MEDIUM PIZZA)

This is a very clever way of making pizza that little bit more healthy by cutting out refined carbohydrates and upping your veg intake at the same time. Add your favourite toppings, like ham, pepperoni, artichokes, olives and jalapeños, and serve with a big green salad on the side. Kids love it too, especially if you get them to put their own toppings on. They don't even suspect that it's cauliflower that they're eating! And the mozzarella provides lots of calcium-rich protein to aid muscle recovery after an active day.

FOR THE BASE
1 medium cauliflower
½ tsp dried oregano
1 egg, beaten
25g grated Parmesan cheese
50g mozzarella cheese, very finely chopped
Olive oil
Sea salt and freshly ground black pepper

FOR THE TOPPING
3 tbsp tomato passata
2 chestnut mushrooms, sliced
1 thyme sprig, leaves only
75g mozzarella cheese, finely sliced

CONTINUED OVERLEAF

PER SERVING	
KCAL	405
FAT (g)	27.0
SATURATES (g)	13.0
CARBS (g)	11.0
SUGARS (g)	8.0
FIBRE (g)	6.0
PROTEIN (g)	26.0
SALT (g)	0.99

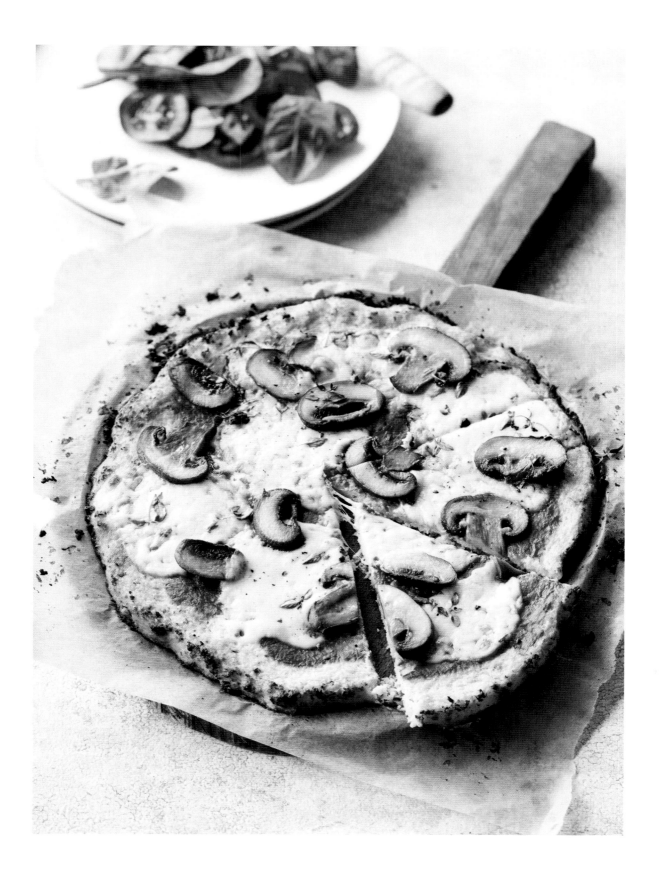

CONTINUED FROM PAGE 244

1. Preheat the oven to 220°C/gas 7.

2. Break the cauliflower into florets and put them into a food processor, then blitz until they resemble breadcrumbs.

3. Put the cauliflower crumbs into a microwave-proof bowl and cover with cling film, leaving a little gap. Cook on full power in the microwave for 6 minutes (see below). Remove and uncover, allowing the steam to escape and the crumbs to cool.

4. Place a baking tray or pizza stone in the oven to heat up.

5. Put the cooked cauliflower on to a clean tea towel or piece of muslin. Draw the tea towel/muslin up around the cauliflower and twist and squeeze until all the moisture has come out.

6. Put the cauliflower into a mixing bowl with the oregano, egg, cheeses and a pinch of salt and pepper and mix together well.

7. Place a large piece of greaseproof paper on a chopping board and rub with a little olive oil. Turn out the cauliflower mixture on to the paper and shape it into a round pizza base about 1cm thick. Rub the top of the pizza base with a little more olive oil.

8. Carefully lift the base, still on the paper, on to the preheated baking tray or pizza stone, then bake in the oven for 8–12 minutes, until golden and crisp.

9. Remove from the oven and cover the top with the passata, using the back of a spoon to spread it out. Scatter with the sliced mushrooms and thyme leaves, then top with the sliced mozzarella and a sprinkle of salt and pepper.

10. Return the pizza to the oven for 5–7 minutes, until the cheese has melted and started to colour. Slice and serve while hot.

HOW TO COOK THE CAULIFLOWER CRUMBS
If you don't have a microwave, steam, boil or bake the crumbs for 5–6 minutes until tender. The only difference is that you will have to work a bit harder to extract all the water in step 5.

BARBECUED SPATCHCOCK POUSSIN WITH ROASTED CORN SALAD

SERVES 4

I love to barbecue and over my many years of firing up the coals, I have learnt that spatchcocking birds really is the best way to cook them evenly. It isn't hard to do (see below) but you can also get your butcher to do it for you. I have given instructions for oven-cooking, too, just in case the British weather lets you down.

4 poussins, spatchcocked
4 whole corn on the cob, husks removed
Juice of 1 lime
1½ tsp chipotle paste
1 tbsp maple syrup
2 tbps olive oil
1 red pepper, deseeded and diced
1 small red onion, peeled and finely diced
3–4 coriander sprigs, stalks chopped,
   leaves reserved
1 x 400g tin black beans, aduki beans
   or pinto beans, drained and rinsed
Sea salt and freshly ground black pepper

FOR THE MARINADE
1 tbsp olive oil
1 small onion, peeled and finely diced
2 garlic cloves, peeled and finely chopped
1 tsp smoked paprika
2 tbsp tomato purée
2 tbsp maple syrup
2 tsp Worcestershire sauce
1 tbsp balsamic vinegar
½–1 tbsp soy sauce, to taste

CONTINUED OVERLEAF

HOW TO SPATCHCOCK A BIRD
To spatchcock a poussin, turn it breast side down with the legs towards you and, using sturdy kitchen scissors, cut along either side of the backbone and remove it. Open the bird out and turn it over so you can flatten it out with your hand.

PER SERVING	
KCAL	829
FAT (g)	47.0
SATURATES (g)	11.0
CARBS (g)	34.0
SUGARS (g)	18.0
FIBRE (g)	13.0
PROTEIN (g)	59.0
SALT (g)	1.16

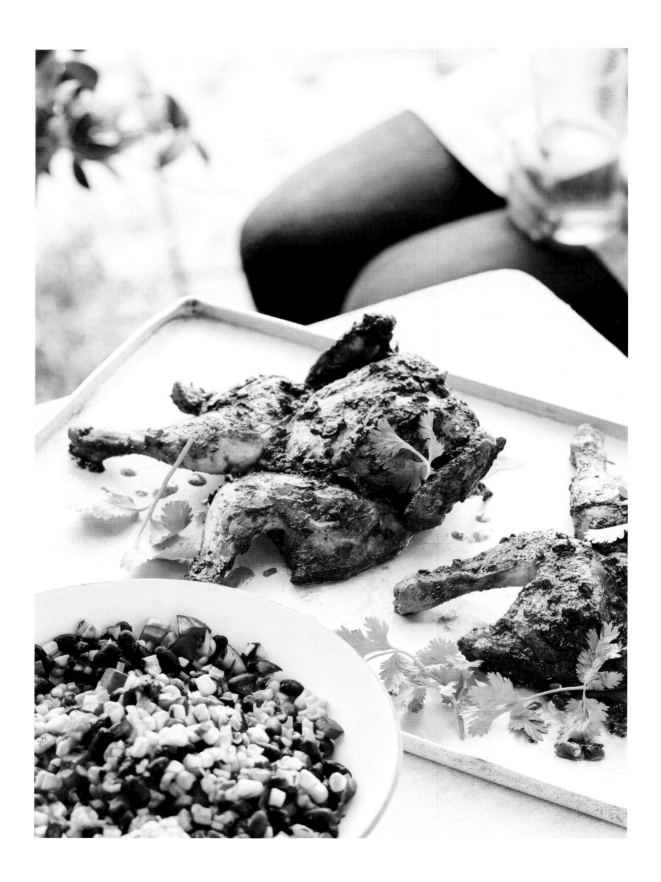

CONTINUED FROM PAGE 247

1. To make the marinade, place a small saucepan over a medium heat and add the olive oil. Once hot, sauté the onion with a pinch of salt for 5 minutes, until softened.

2. Add the garlic and continue to cook for 1 minute, then add the remaining marinade ingredients. Stir well and simmer gently for 5–6 minutes. Taste and adjust the seasoning as necessary, adding more soy sauce for a more savoury flavour. Leave to cool.

3. When the marinade has cooled down, put the poussins into a suitable container and pour over the marinade. Cover the dish with cling film and put it into the fridge for at least an hour, or up to 2 days.

4. When ready to cook, light the barbecue or preheat the oven to 180°C/gas 4 and remove the poussins from the fridge to let them come up to room temperature.

5. To barbecue, when the coals are medium hot put the poussins on the grill for 20 minutes, or until cooked through, turning after 10 minutes.

6. To oven cook, put the marinated poussins on a roasting tray, breast side up, and into the preheated oven. Roast for 30–35 minutes, until cooked through, basting occasionally. (If the extremities of the poussins look like they might burn, cover with a piece of kitchen foil for the remainder of the cooking time.)

7. Meanwhile, heat a griddle pan or grill until very hot and cook the corn on all sides until lightly charred. This will take about 7–10 minutes. (To barbecue the corn, place them on the grill before the chicken while the coals are still very hot.)

8. While the corn is cooking, put the lime juice, chipotle paste, maple syrup, olive oil and a pinch of salt and pepper into a jam jar with a tight-fitting lid and shake until combined.

9. Remove the kernels from the cob by placing the cobs on their ends on a chopping board and running a sharp knife along the cob. Put the kernels into a large mixing bowl.

10. Add the red pepper, red onion, coriander stalks and beans and pour in the dressing. Toss well to make sure everything is coated, then taste and adjust the seasoning as necessary.

11. Once the poussins are cooked, remove from the oven and leave to rest for 5–10 minutes. Sprinkle with the coriander leaves, and serve with the corn salad and lots of napkins!

CELEBRATION SIDE OF SALMON WITH LEMON AND WASABI
SERVES 6–8

This recipe is ideal for a post-race party – if you've got the energy to cook it, that is! It's very easy to put together and the fish looks after itself once it's in the oven. The added bonus is that it is delicious served hot, warm, at room temperature or even cold, so if you get distracted when it's out of the oven it won't spoil. Better still, get someone else to cook it for you while you rest your aching muscles . . . Serve it with new potatoes, green salad and lots of home-made mayonnaise.

1 x 1.5kg side of salmon, skin on, descaled and pin-boned
Juice of 1½ lemons
2 tsp wasabi paste or powder
2 tbsp Worcestershire sauce
2 tbsp olive oil
Sea salt and freshly ground black pepper

TO SERVE
Rocket leaves
Lemon wedges

1. Preheat the oven to 200°C/gas 6.

2. Place the side of salmon, skin side down, in a large roasting tin lined with greaseproof paper.

3. Mix together the lemon juice, wasabi, Worcestershire sauce and olive oil until completely combined, then season with salt and pepper.

4. Pour the mixture over the salmon, making sure the sides of the salmon have some of the marinade on them as well as the top.

5. Put the tray into the preheated oven and bake the salmon for 20–25 minutes, until just cooked through.

6. Remove from the oven and allow to rest for a few minutes. Scatter over some rocket leaves and serve with lemon wedges.

PER SERVING	
KCAL	525
FAT (g)	34.0
SATURATES (g)	6.0
CARBS (g)	2.0
SUGARS (g)	1.0
FIBRE (g)	0.0
PROTEIN (g)	52.0
SALT (g)	0.44

FEEDING A CROWD
You can scale this recipe up if you are catering for larger numbers. You should be able to fit two 1.5kg sides of salmon head to toe in a large roasting tin, or you can use two roasting tins and swap shelves halfway through cooking. Two 1.5kg sides of salmon should feed 12–15 people.

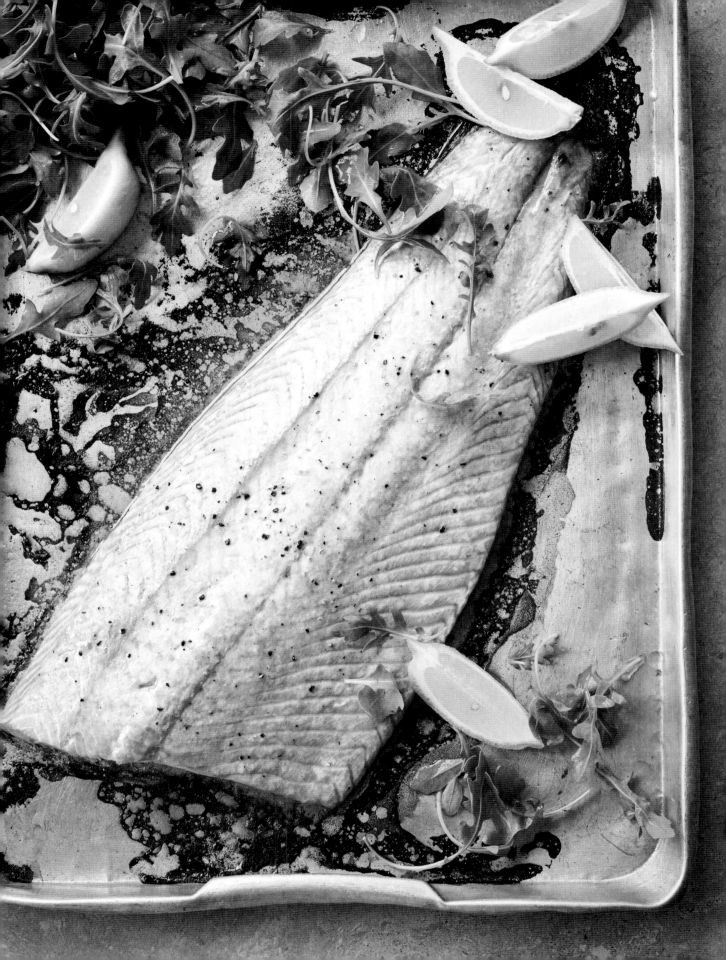

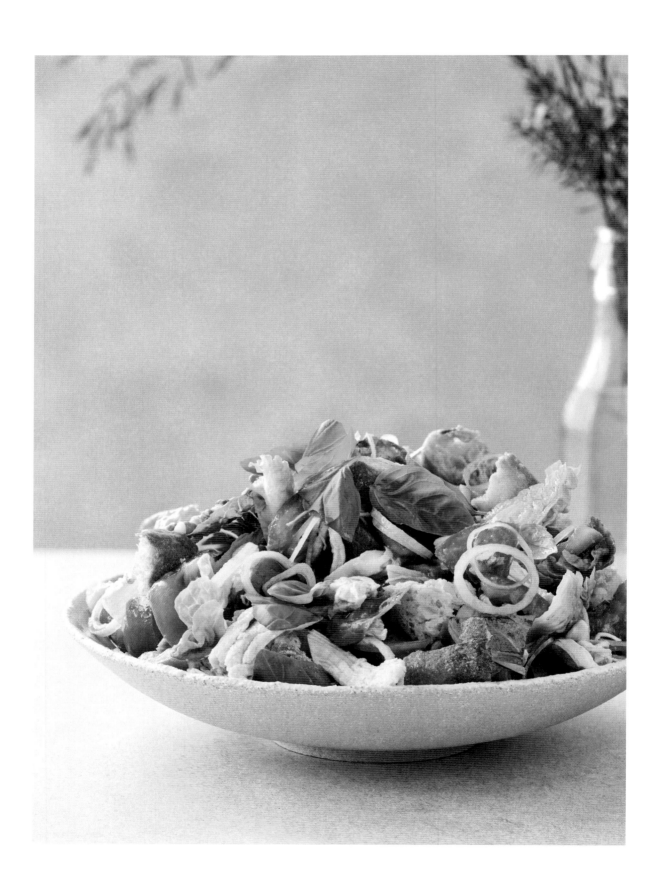

PANZANELLA WITH POACHED CHICKEN

SERVES 4

Panzanella is an Italian bread and tomato salad with a strong anchovy dressing that will really liven up a simple poached chicken supper. As always when serving tomatoes, make sure you choose the ripest you can find, as they will have much more flavour and sweetness than unripe ones. Be careful not to boil the chicken breasts, and always leave them in the stock to cool because removing them from the liquid while hot will dry them out.

1 litre chicken stock
4 chicken breasts, skin removed
½ large ciabatta loaf
40ml olive oil
2½ tbsp red wine vinegar
2 large shallots, peeled and cut into thin rounds
1 rosemary sprig, leaves only
2 anchovy fillets, drained and finely chopped
4 large, ripe tomatoes
3 baby gem lettuces, leaves separated and washed
1 bunch of basil, leaves only
Sea salt and freshly ground black pepper

1. Preheat the oven to 180°C/gas 4.

2. Put the chicken stock into a saucepan and bring to the boil. Add the chicken breasts, then reduce the heat to its lowest setting and cover with a lid. Cook the chicken for 10 minutes, then turn the heat off completely and leave the breasts to cool in the stock until you are ready to serve.

3. Cut the ciabatta into 3cm chunks and scatter them over a baking tray. Place in the oven for 10 minutes, until the bread has crisped up. Remove the tray from the oven and leave to cool.

4. Pour the oil and red wine vinegar into a bowl and add the shallot rings, rosemary leaves and chopped anchovies.

5. Place a sieve or colander over the bowl, then roughly chop the tomatoes into 12 large chunks per tomato and place in the colander. Roughly crush the tomatoes with the back of a wooden spoon to release some of their juice.

6. When ready to serve, tip the tomatoes from the colander into a large serving bowl, then add the toasted bread and baby gem lettuce leaves.

7. Remove the chicken breasts from the stock and tear them into large chunks with a knife and fork, then add them to the salad bowl.

8. Whisk together the dressing ingredients with the tomato juice, season with salt and pepper and pour into the bowl. Toss everything together and sprinkle over the basil leaves before serving.

PER SERVING	
KCAL	469
FAT (g)	14.0
SATURATES (g)	3.0
CARBS (g)	30.0
SUGARS (g)	9.0
FIBRE (g)	7.0
PROTEIN (g)	52.0
SALT (g)	1.52

GARLIC AND PARSLEY POT ROAST GUINEA FOWL

SERVES 4

To me, this is the perfect evening meal after a winter race or heavy training session. It is so warming and restorative and full of the proteins and complex carbohydrates your body needs when it has pushed itself to the limit. Having spent time cooking in France, I really love guinea fowl, especially pot-roasted in this way, but you could easily make this with chicken too.

1½ tbsp olive oil
1 large guinea fowl
1 onion, peeled and diced
1 carrot, diced
2 celery sticks, diced
1 bay leaf
Small bunch of parsley, leaves picked
    and stalks tied in a bundle with chefs' string
4 garlic cloves, peeled and sliced
100ml dry sherry
500ml chicken stock
150g Puy lentils
Squeeze of lemon juice, to taste
Sea salt and freshly ground black pepper

1. Preheat the oven to 180°C/gas 4.

2. Place a large casserole dish with a lid over a medium heat and add 1 tablespoon of the olive oil. Season the guinea fowl with salt and pepper and, when the oil is hot, place breast side down in the casserole dish. Leave for 3–4 minutes to brown, then turn and continue browning until golden all over. Remove and put to one side.

3. Add the remaining olive oil to the casserole and add the onion, carrot, celery, bay leaf and parsley stalks with a pinch of salt and pepper. Stir, cover with the lid and cook for 6–8 minutes, until the onion is soft. Remove the lid, add the garlic and cook for a further 1–2 minutes until aromatic and soft.

4. Add the sherry to deglaze the pan, scraping up any bits from the bottom, and allow to bubble for 2 minutes.

CONTINUED OVERLEAF

PER SERVING	
KCAL	500
FAT (g)	16.0
SATURATES (g)	4.0
CARBS (g)	23.0
SUGARS (g)	4.0
FIBRE (g)	7.0
PROTEIN (g)	54.0
SALT (g)	0.67

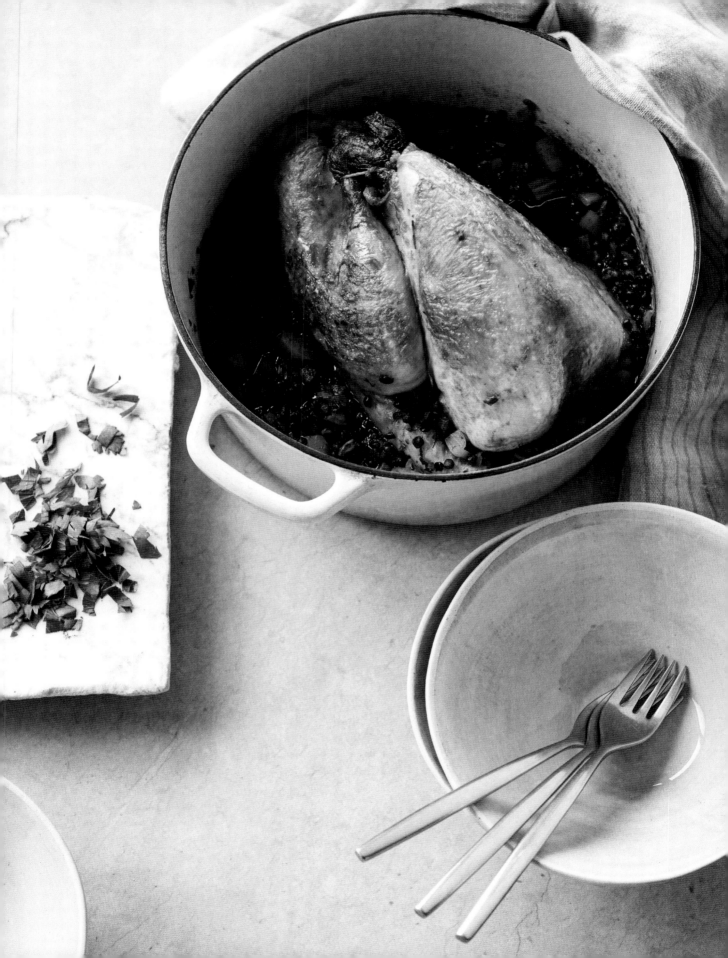

CONTINUED FROM PAGE 254

5. Add the chicken stock and the lentils and stir, then put the guinea fowl, breast side up, back into the casserole dish, pushing it down into the lentils so that the liquid and the lentils rise up around the bird.

6. Put the lid on and transfer to the preheated oven for 50 minutes. Remove the lid and give the lentils a stir, then put back into the oven and cook for a further 10 minutes uncovered, to colour the skin on the breast a little more.

7. Remove from the oven and take the guinea fowl out of the casserole. Put it on a board to rest for 5 minutes.

8. Meanwhile, give the lentils a stir and taste. Add a squeeze of lemon and a little salt and pepper if needed, and taste again to check the seasoning. Remove the parsley stalks and bay leaf.

9. Roughly chop the parsley leaves, add to the dish and stir through.

10. Joint the guinea fowl (see below) and put the pieces back into the casserole dish with the lentils. Pour any juices that run off while carving into the lentils.

11. Bring the casserole dish to the table for people to help themselves, and serve with seasonal green vegetables.

HOW TO JOINT A COOKED GUINEA FOWL
Cut through the skin that joins the legs to the breast and pull the legs away from the body until they come free at the joint. Using a very sharp knife, cut down between the thigh and the drumstick to separate them. To remove the breasts, run the knife along the breastbone, pulling the breast away as you cut.

SPICED KOFTAS WITH BULGUR WHEAT SALAD

SERVES 4

All the flavours of the Middle East and North Africa converge in this protein-rich banquet. It is a particularly good choice for a recovery meal because everything can be made in advance, with only the grilling of the koftas to be done on the night, leaving you to enjoy a well-deserved sit down before tucking into a delicious restorative feast.

2 tbsp olive oil
2 small red onions, peeled and diced
1 garlic clove, peeled and diced
1 x 400g tin cannellini beans, drained and rinsed
1 x 400g tin chopped tomatoes
1–2 tsp harissa paste, to taste
500ml chicken or vegetable stock
250g dried bulgur wheat
125g lean lamb mince (less than 10% fat)
175g lean turkey mince (less than 2% fat)
1 egg

75g fresh breadcrumbs
1½ tsp ground cinnamon
1½ tsp ground cumin
Large bunch of parsley, roughly chopped
Large bunch of mint, leaves roughly chopped
Juice of 1 lemon
Sea salt and freshly ground black pepper

TO SERVE
Flatbreads
0% fat Greek yoghurt

CONTINUED OVERLEAF

PER SERVING	
KCAL	561
FAT (g)	12.0
SATURATES (g)	3.0
CARBS (g)	67.0
SUGARS (g)	8.0
FIBRE (g)	16.0
PROTEIN (g)	37.0
SALT (g)	1.04

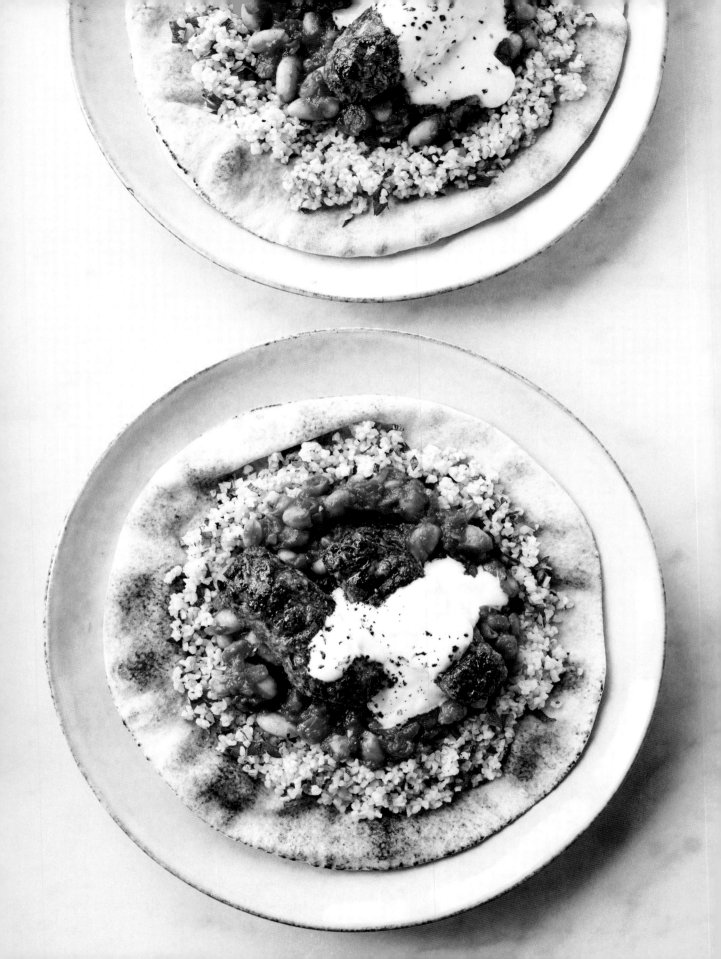

CONTINUED FROM PAGE 257

1. Place a saucepan over a medium–high heat and add 1 tablespoon of the olive oil. When hot, add half the chopped onion and the garlic and sweat for 5 minutes. Add the cannellini beans and chopped tomatoes along with half a tin of water. Bring the liquid to the boil, then reduce to a simmer for 10 minutes.

2. Remove the pan from the heat, stir in the harissa paste and season with a little salt and pepper.

3. Bring the chicken stock to the boil and tip the bulgur wheat into a large bowl. When the stock is boiling, pour it over the bulgur, cover with cling film and leave to sit for a minimum of 10 minutes.

4. Meanwhile, using clean hands, mix the two minced meats with the egg, breadcrumbs, cinnamon, cumin, the remaining chopped red onion and a good pinch of salt and pepper. Work the mixture until it comes together, then shape into 8 small sausage shapes.

5. Heat the grill to high and, when hot, grill the koftas for 8–10 minutes, turning a few times. Make sure they are fully cooked through by cutting into a thick kofta to check the meat is no longer pink in the middle.

6. Turn the grill off and leave the meat to rest in the warmth of the grill.

7. Remove the cling film from the bulgur wheat, pour in the remaining tablespoon of olive oil and fluff the grains with a fork. Add the parsley, mint and lemon juice, season with a good pinch of salt and pepper, and stir.

8. Serve the koftas with the rich beans, bulgur salad, flatbread and a big dollop of Greek yoghurt.

BAVETTE STEAK WITH ROSEMARY CHIMICHURRI

SERVES 4

Bavette steak, also known as 'skirt', is cut from the flank of the cow and because it is less tender than rump steak, it is often marinated or slow-cooked. When it is cooked on a griddle like this, it is vital to keep the cooking time down so that it is served medium-rare and then to carve it against the grain to keep it from being chewy. You will probably have to order a whole piece of bavette from your butcher but it is definitely worth it. This can get very smoky, so turn the extractor fan to max, open the windows and get ready to silence the smoke alarm. It's ideal for barbecuing in the great outdoors, too.

Large bunch of parsley, finely chopped
Small bunch of oregano, leaves finely chopped
3 garlic cloves, peeled and crushed
2 rosemary sprigs, leaves finely chopped
1 red chilli, deseeded and finely chopped
35ml red wine vinegar
30ml rapeseed oil
1kg piece of bavette steak
4 Portobello mushrooms, brushed clean
  and cut into thick slices
12 whole cherry tomatoes on the vine
Sea salt and freshly ground black pepper
Watercress, to serve

1. Mix together the parsley, oregano, garlic, rosemary, chilli, red wine vinegar and a third of the oil. Season with a little salt and pepper then leave to infuse for approximately 2 hours.

2. When ready to cook, heat a large griddle pan over a high heat.

3. Brush the steak on both sides with the remaining oil, then, when the griddle is smoking hot, carefully put it on to the pan and fry for 4 minutes on each side. Remove the steak, wrap in tin foil and leave to rest.

4. Put the sliced mushrooms on to the griddle in a single layer and cook for 2 minutes on each side. Take the mushrooms off the griddle, then add the tomatoes and cook for approximately 2 minutes as well.

5. Carve the steak against the grain into long, thin slices and arrange the slices on a serving platter. Drizzle with a generous amount of chimichurri sauce and serve with the mushrooms, tomatoes and watercress.

PER SERVING	
KCAL	554
FAT (g)	32.0
SATURATES (g)	10.0
CARBS (g)	4.0
SUGARS (g)	4.0
FIBRE (g)	4.0
PROTEIN (g)	60.0
SALT (g)	0.45

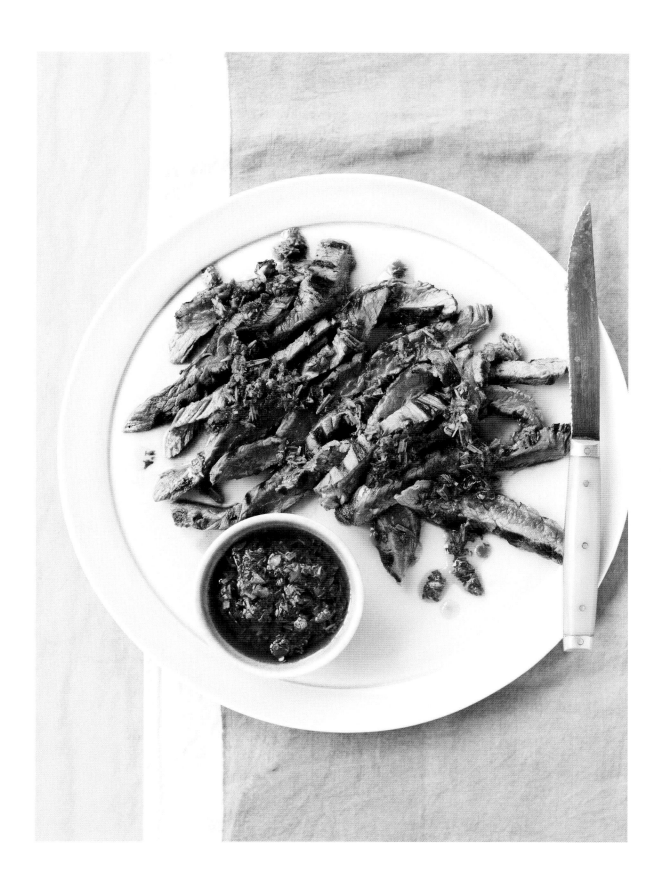

HIGH-ENERGY SNACKS AND WELL-DESERVED TREATS

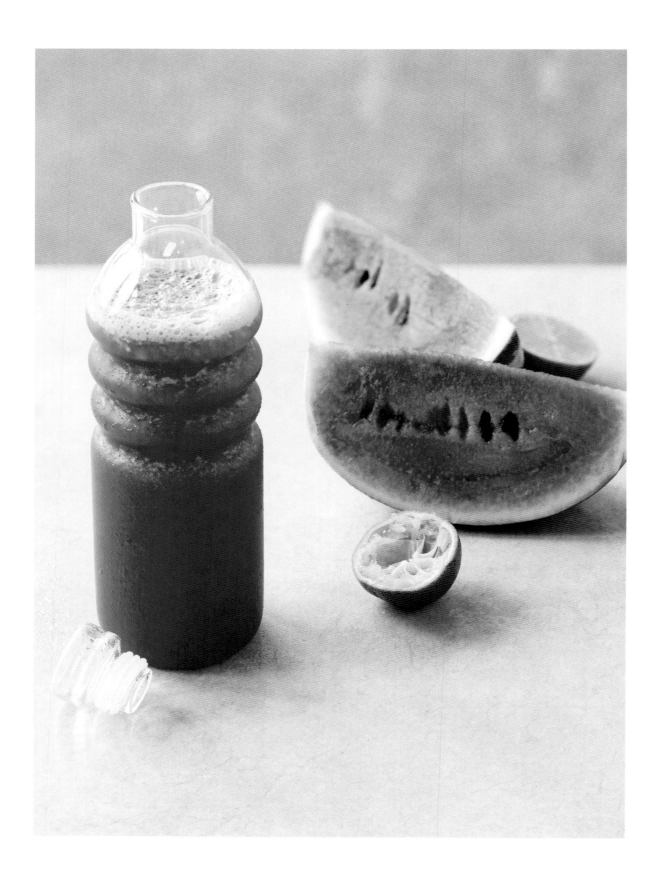

WATERMELON COOLER

SERVES 6

What you drink before, during and after exercise is just as important as what you eat, and this easy juice provides excellent hydration as well as instant energy without any free sugars. The pinch of salt isn't essential but it helps replenish the body's sodium levels, which are seriously depleted by sweating over a long period of time.

1kg watermelon flesh (about ½ medium watermelon), cut into chunks
Juice of 1 lime
Pinch of salt

1. Put the watermelon chunks into a blender and blitz until smooth. Add the lime juice and a pinch of salt and blend again.

2. Add 2 handfuls of ice and blend once more until the ice is broken up. If the mixture is very thick then blend in 200ml of cold water.

3. Serve in glasses with extra ice cubes or pour into your water bottle to take with you.

VARIATIONS
You can alter the flavour slightly by adding herbs or a pinch of chilli. Basil works well, as does mint.

PER SERVING	
KCAL	56
FAT (g)	0.3
SATURATES (g)	0.0
CARBS (g)	12.0
SUGARS (g)	10.0
FIBRE (g)	1.0
PROTEIN (g)	1.0
SALT (g)	0.9

PITTA CRISPS WITH RED PEPPER DIP

SERVES 4

Making your own pitta crisps is both healthier and cheaper than buying ready-made crisps when you're having dips. They are the perfect accompaniment for snacks like the Minted Baba Ganoush on page 95 and the Smoky Flageolet Bean Houmous on page 94 and are an easy way to add more carbs to soups and salads when you need them. The dip is very versatile, too – it's delicious with seafood such as prawns or grilled squid and is also great on pasta.

4 large wholemeal pitta breads
1 garlic clove, peeled and crushed
½ tsp dried mixed herbs
2 tbsp olive oil
Sea salt

FOR THE RED PEPPER DIP
350g roasted red peppers in brine, drained
1½ tsp sherry vinegar
75g flaked almonds
2 tbsp olive oil
Sea salt and freshly ground black pepper

1. Preheat the oven to 180°C/gas 4.

2. Cut each pitta bread into 8 triangles, then divide each triangle into 2 thinner triangles and place them in a single layer on two baking trays.

3. Mix together the crushed garlic, dried herbs and olive oil. Brush each side of the triangles with a little of the mixture and sprinkle with a pinch of salt. Put the trays into the preheated oven and bake for 3–4 minutes, then turn the triangles over, removing any thinner pieces that are already crisp. Return the tray to the oven and cook for a further 2–3 minutes, until all the triangles are golden brown and crisp. Remove from the oven and leave to cool.

4. For the red pepper dip, put all the ingredients into a food processor and blitz until smooth, then season with salt and pepper. If the consistency is a bit thick, add a tablespoon of water and blitz again.

5. Serve the pitta crisps and some fresh crudités with the dip as a great on-the-go lunch or a snack for sharing with friends. Any leftover dip can be stored covered in the fridge for up to 3 days.

PER SERVING	
KCAL	386
FAT (g)	22.0
SATURATES (g)	3.0
CARBS (g)	32.0
SUGARS (g)	3.0
FIBRE (g)	4.0
PROTEIN (g)	12.0
SALT (g)	1.95

HOW TO STORE PITTA CRISPS
The pitta crisps can be stored in an airtight container for up to a week. If they need crisping up before eating, put them into an oven preheated to 150°C/gas 2 for 5 minutes.

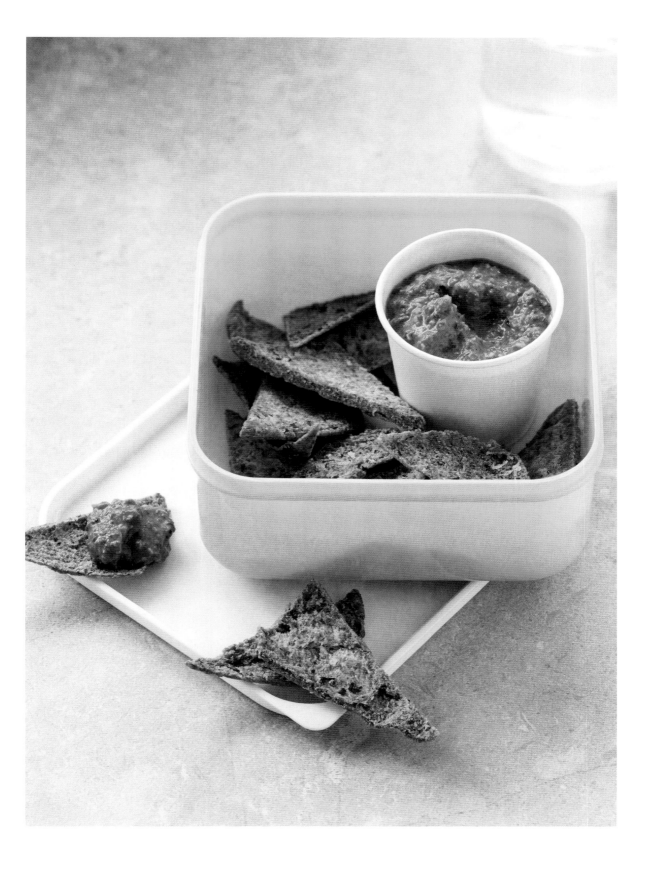

SEED AND NUT 'GRANOLA' BARS

MAKES 18 BARS

Granola bars are my go-to snacks when I'm training for a triathlon. They're easy to make, perfect for carrying around and they give me everything I need to be able to perform at my absolute best. The dates act as the glue that binds everything together, but you can vary the other ingredients depending on what you like or have in the cupboard. These are also good for camping trips, picnics and packed lunches.

200g dates, pitted
2 tbsp nut butter e.g. peanut, cashew or almond butter
2 tbsp coconut oil
100g rolled oats
75g almonds
75g Brazil nuts
2 tbsp mixed seeds, e.g. sunflower, pumpkin and linseed
50g puffed brown rice (optional)

1. Place the dates in a food processor with 4 tablespoons of hot water and blend until smooth. If the mixture is a bit lumpy, add hot water 1 tablespoon at a time, blending between additions until you have a smooth paste.

2. Add the nut butter and coconut oil and blend until combined, then add the oats, almonds and Brazil nuts and pulse briefly to mix through but not break down completely.

3. Gently stir in the mixed seeds and puffed rice, if using, by hand.

4. Line a brownie tin (approximately 25cm x 18cm) with greaseproof paper and pour the mixture into the tin. Flatten the surface until roughly level.

5. Cover with cling film and put into the fridge to chill until completely firm (about an hour).

6. Cut into squares or bar shapes, and keep in the fridge for up to a week.

PER BAR	
KCAL	139
FAT (g)	8.0
SATURATES (g)	2.0
CARBS (g)	12.0
SUGARS (g)	8.0
FIBRE (g)	2.0
PROTEIN (g)	3.0
SALT (g)	0.01

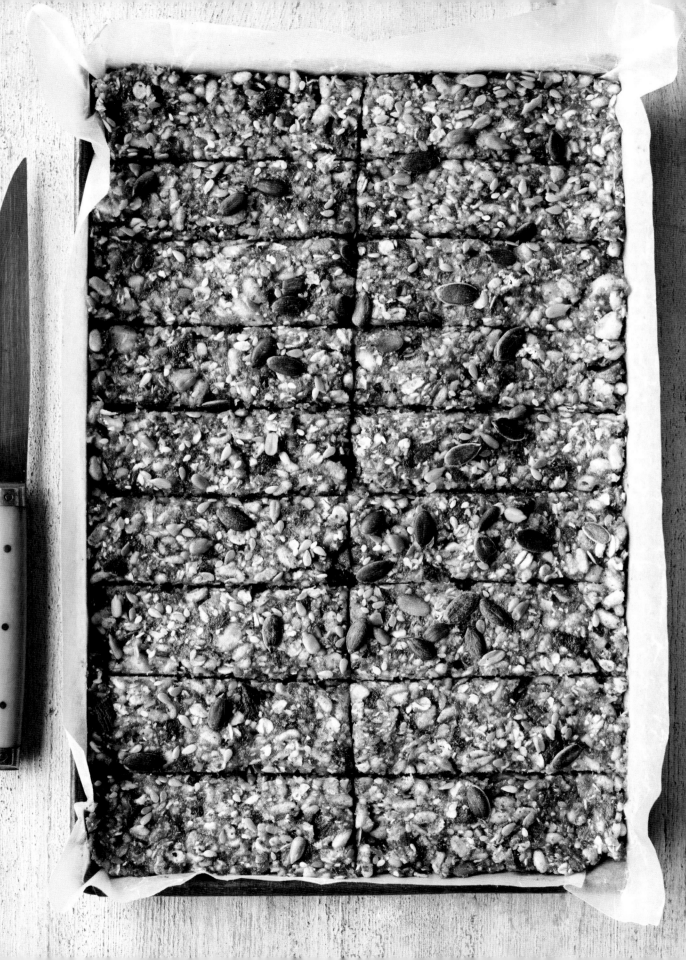

RAW CHOCOLATE MILKSHAKE

SERVES 4

If you get cravings for chocolate milkshake, make it as natural as possible by blitzing up your own with almond milk, cacao nibs and dates. Yes, it's really sweet, but the fibre in the dates and the natural fats in the cacao powder mean the energy is slow-releasing and won't play havoc with your blood sugar levels after consuming. Swap the almond milk for cow's milk if you need extra protein after a tough workout or competition.

1 litre unsweetened almond milk
8 tbsp cacao powder
8–12 dates, stoned
Maple syrup (optional)

1. Put the almond milk, cacao powder and dates into a blender and blitz until smooth.

2. Taste and add a little maple syrup, if needed.

3. Add a handful of ice cubes to the milkshake and blend again to chill completely.

4. Pour into four glasses and serve with a straw.

PER SERVING	
KCAL	154
FAT (g)	6.0
SATURATES (g)	2.0
CARBS (g)	17.0
SUGARS (g)	14.0
FIBRE (g)	7.0
PROTEIN (g)	6.0
SALT (g)	0.33

VARIATION
You can also add bananas and nut butters to this milkshake.

MUESLI ENERGY BITES

MAKES 14 BITES

These oat, fruit and nut energy balls are the equivalent of eating a bowl of muesli in a couple of bites. They are full of easy-access energy when you need it most, and are brilliant for when you don't have time for breakfast or for a quick boost before a workout or run. We always have a version of these or the Raw Choco Treats (see page 273) in the fridge so everyone in the family can help themselves when they need to.

100g unsweetened peanut butter,
   smooth or crunchy
3 tbsp runny honey
125g rolled oats
150g raisins
50g walnuts, very finely chopped

1. Mix together the peanut butter and honey in a large mixing bowl until combined. Pour in the oats, raisins and finely chopped walnuts and mix really well, until everything is coated in the peanut butter honey mixture.

2. Place the mixture in the fridge for 20 minutes to firm up a little.

3. Once firm, remove from the fridge and, using your hands, form the mixture into balls about 3–4cm wide, squeezing the mixture together to make it stick. Place the balls on a tray and chill in the fridge for at least an hour, to set.

4. Transfer to an airtight container and store in the fridge or somewhere cool until needed. They will keep for 1–2 weeks in the fridge.

HOW TO MAKE MUESLI BISCUITS
To turn these bites into crisp biscuits, put the balls on to a baking tray lined with baking paper and press into flat circles. Put the tray into an oven preheated to 160°C/gas 3 and bake for 10–12 minutes until golden and crisp on the outside and chewy on the inside.

PER ENERGY BITE	
KCAL	150
FAT (g)	7.0
SATURATES (g)	1.0
CARBS (g)	17.0
SUGARS (g)	11.0
FIBRE (g)	2.0
PROTEIN (g)	4.0
SALT (g)	0.08

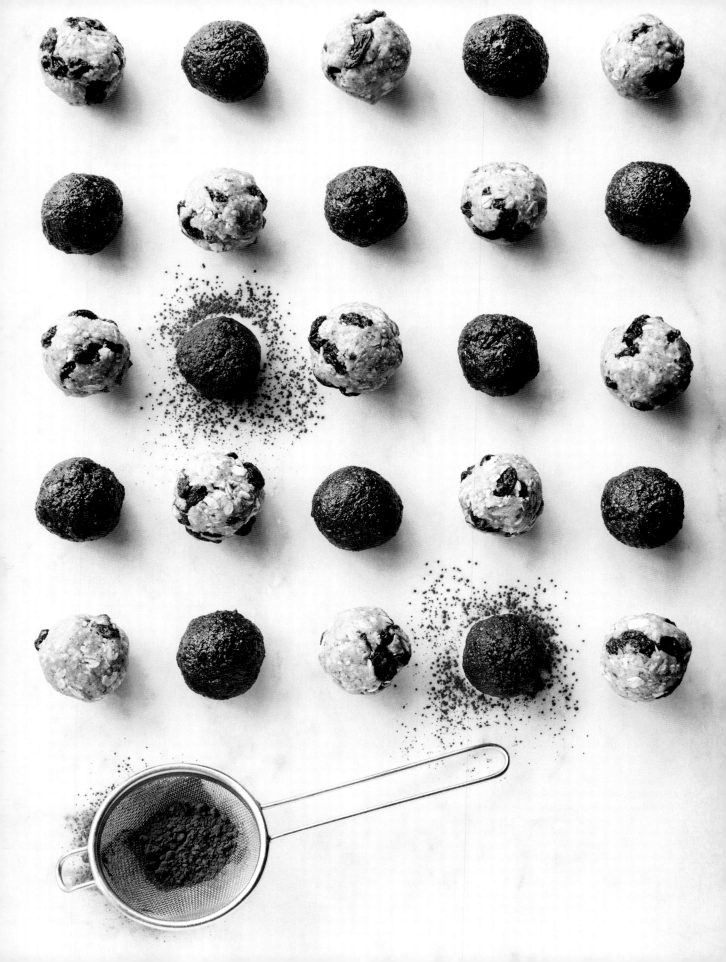

RAW CHOCO TREATS

MAKES 14 TREATS

Tana has given me her secret recipe for these incredible chocolate snacks, which are also known as 'bliss balls', apparently. You can add any nuts or seeds that you like or roll them in desiccated coconut for a bit of crunch. They make a really good pre-exercise snack as well as a general energy boost in the middle of a busy day.

75g stoned dates
2 tbsp coconut oil
1 tbsp almond butter
75g almonds
3 tbsp cacao powder,
    plus a little for dusting

1. Put the dates and coconut oil into a food processor and blend until a smooth paste has formed.

2. Add the almond butter and blend to mix, then add the almonds and blend again until they are finely chopped.

3. Finally, add the cacao powder and blend until the mixture starts to stick together and all the ingredients are finely chopped.

4. Using a teaspoon, take 1 heaped spoonful of the mixture and roll it between your hands into a ball. Place on a plate or tray and repeat with the remaining mixture. Dust with a little extra cacao powder, then cover the balls with cling film and put into the fridge to firm up for at least 2 hours.

5. Once firm, transfer them to an airtight container and keep them in the fridge for up to 2 weeks.

HOW TO MAKE AHEAD
Make a big batch of these balls and freeze the spares. They taste delicious straight from the freezer, or can be defrosted in the fridge until ready to eat.

PER TREAT	
KCAL	78
FAT (g)	6.0
SATURATES (g)	2.0
CARBS (g)	4.0
SUGARS (g)	4.0
FIBRE (g)	1.0
PROTEIN (g)	2.0
SALT (g)	0.01

FIG ROLLS

MAKES 16 ROLLS

It would be impossible to calculate how many fig rolls I have eaten in my lifetime . . . Let's just agree that it's a lot! It started when my mum used to put them in my lunchbox when I was a kid and now, 40 years later, they are one of my favourite training snacks. For me, a home-made snack in the middle of a triathlon gives me more than just a physical energy boost, it lifts my spirits in a way that an isotonic gel or shop-bought muesli bar never could.

300g soft figs, trimmed and roughly chopped
225g wholemeal flour, plus a little
   extra for dusting
1 tsp baking powder
70g coconut oil
½ tsp ground cinnamon
1 egg
70ml semi-skimmed milk, plus a little
   extra for brushing
2 pinches of Demerara sugar

1. Put the chopped figs into a saucepan with 250ml water and bring to the boil. Cover with a lid and simmer for 15 minutes until the figs are very soft. Keep an eye on the pan to make sure it doesn't cook dry.

2. Remove the pan from the heat and, using the back of a wooden spoon, crush the larger pieces to break them up. Tip the figs into a bowl and leave them to cool completely.

3. Put the wholemeal flour, baking powder, coconut oil and ground cinnamon into a food processor and blitz until the ingredients are fully incorporated.

4. Add the egg and milk and pulse until the pastry comes together.

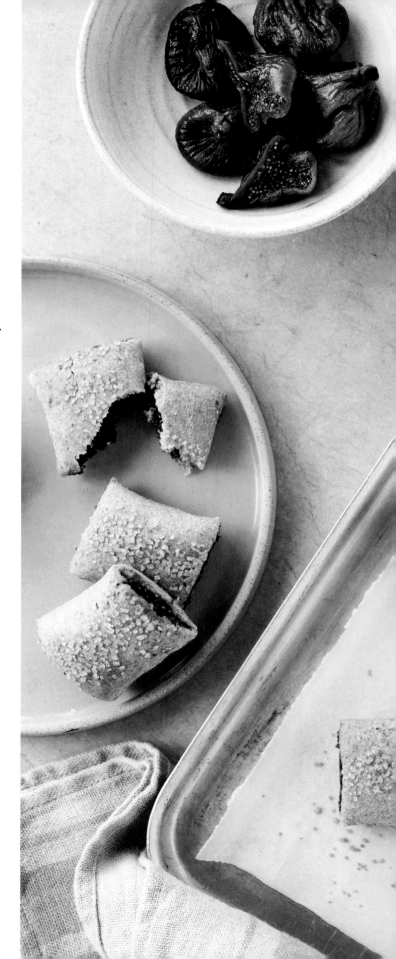

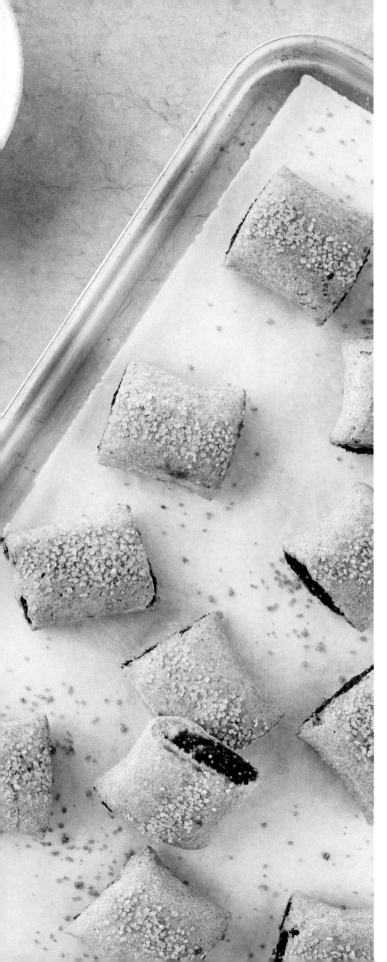

5. Tip the pastry on to a clean work surface and knead for 30 seconds before wrapping in cling film and leaving to rest for 20 minutes.

6. When ready to cook, preheat the oven to 210°C/gas 6.

7. Unwrap the pastry and cut it into 2 equal-sized pieces. Dust a clean surface with a little wholemeal flour then roll out the first half into a rectangle roughly 30cm x 11cm in size.

8. Spoon half of the fig mixture in a line across the middle of the rectangle. Roll one side of the pastry over the other, gently pushing to join the seam. Trim any excess pastry, then repeat the process with the other piece of pastry.

9. Brush the rolls with milk then sprinkle with Demerara sugar and cut each one into 8 equal-sized pieces. Place the pieces on to a baking tray lined with baking paper, then place in the preheated oven for 15 minutes.

10. Remove the tray from the oven and allow the fig rolls to cool completely before eating.

HOW TO MAKE THE PASTRY
This pastry really needs to be made in a food processor to incorporate the coconut oil. It can be done by hand but it takes a very long time!

PER FIG ROLL	
KCAL	140
FAT (g)	5.0
SATURATES (g)	4.0
CARBS (g)	19.0
SUGARS (g)	9.0
FIBRE (g)	3.0
PROTEIN (g)	3.0
SALT (g)	0.12

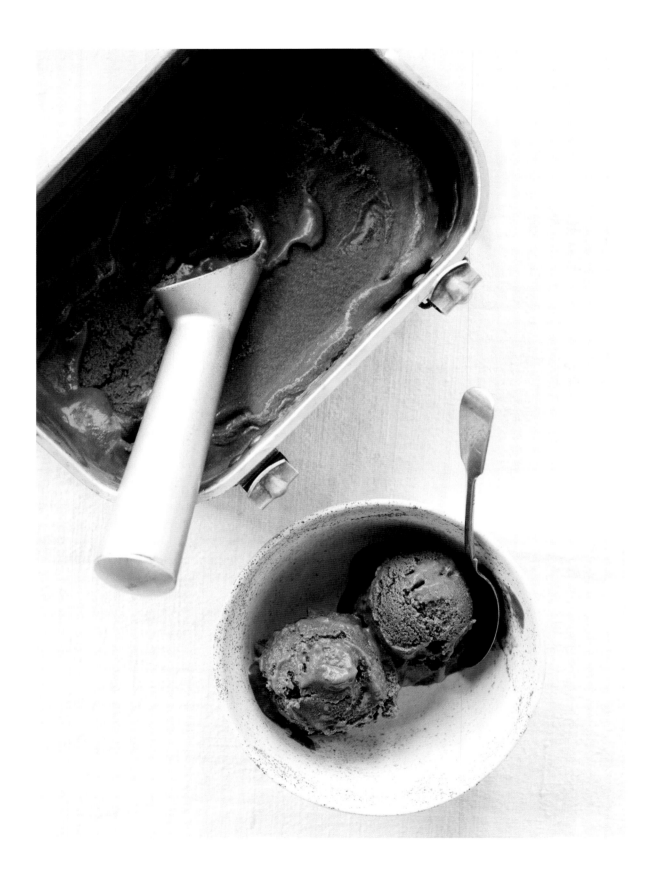

PEANUT BUTTER AND CHOCOLATE ICE CREAM

SERVES 6

This is a variation of the incredibly simple Banana 'Ice Cream' on page 180, with added peanut butter to provide a post-exercise protein hit for tired muscles. The coconut milk makes it even more creamy, and can also restore some of the vital nutrients lost when taking part in strenuous training. It's extremely indulgent but really great when you've earned it.

1 x 400g tin coconut milk
1 large ripe banana, cut into chunks and
    frozen for at least 4 hours
3 tbsp peanut butter, smooth or chunky
2 tbsp cacao powder
Honey or maple syrup (optional)

1. Put the coconut milk and banana into a food processor and blend until smooth, occasionally scraping down the sides.

2. Add the peanut butter and cacao powder and blend until well mixed. Taste and sweeten with honey or maple syrup, if necessary.

3. Pour into a freezer-proof container with a lid and put into the freezer for 2–4 hours, until almost set.

4. Remove from the freezer and blend again, then put back into the container and freeze until set. This should result in a smoother ice cream with fewer ice crystals.

5. To serve, remove from the freezer 20–30 minutes before serving to allow for easy scooping.

VARIATION
If you prefer not to use coconut milk you can make this by simply blending 4 chopped frozen bananas with the peanut butter and the cacao until smooth, then freezing.

PER SERVING	
KCAL	190
FAT (g)	16.0
SATURATES (g)	11.0
CARBS (g)	7.0
SUGARS (g)	5.0
FIBRE (g)	2.0
PROTEIN (g)	4.0
SALT (g)	0.07

CHEESECAKE
IN A JAM JAR
SERVES 4

This is a really indulgent treat for when it's all over
. . . It's almost as naughty as a regular cheesecake,
but the almonds in the base and the Greek yoghurt
mixed into the topping mean that it's a more
nourishing version than the classic; it's full of
protein, calcium and vitamins to support your
muscles and bones after exertion. Putting this
in jam jars makes it very portable, but if you are
staying at home you can use glasses instead.

FOR THE BASE
200g almonds, skins on
3 tbsp coconut oil
2 tbsp coconut sugar or golden caster sugar

FOR THE TOPPING
250g low-fat cream cheese, at room temperature
300g Greek yoghurt
1–2 tbsp coconut sugar, maple syrup
  or runny honey, to taste
1 tbsp lemon juice
1 tbsp vanilla extract
200g frozen blueberries, defrosted
Pinch of salt

1. Toast the almonds in a dry frying pan over a
medium heat for 3–4 minutes, until they smell
nutty and toasted. Leave to cool slightly.

2. Pour the toasted almonds into a food processor
and blitz until finely chopped. Add the coconut oil
and sugar and blend until completely incorporated.

3. Divide the mixture between four small jam jars
and press down to make a firm base. Place the jars
in the fridge to firm up while you make the topping.

4. Put the cream cheese and yoghurt into a mixing
bowl and beat together with a wooden spoon.
Once mixed, add 1 tablespoon of the coconut sugar,
maple syrup or honey, with the lemon juice, vanilla
and a pinch of salt. Mix again and taste, adding the
remaining sugar, honey or maple syrup, if needed.

5. Stir half the blueberries into the topping and
roughly mix so that they aren't completely broken
up but instead give a swirling pattern to the mixture.

6. Remove the jam jars from the fridge and divide the
topping mixture between them, filling each one until
there is a 2cm gap from the top. Tap the bottom of the
jars gently on the work surface to level out the filling.

7. Divide the remaining blueberries between the jars,
making sure you don't over-fill them if you plan to
put the lids on for transportation.

8. Return the jars to the fridge and chill for at least
an hour to firm up.

9. Serve the cheesecakes straight from the fridge
with teaspoons, or put them into a cool bag to take
with you on a picnic.

PER SERVING	
KCAL	638
FAT (g)	46.0
SATURATES (g)	16.0
CARBS (g)	28.0
SUGARS (g)	22.0
FIBRE (g)	2.0
PROTEIN (g)	24.0
SALT (g)	0.55

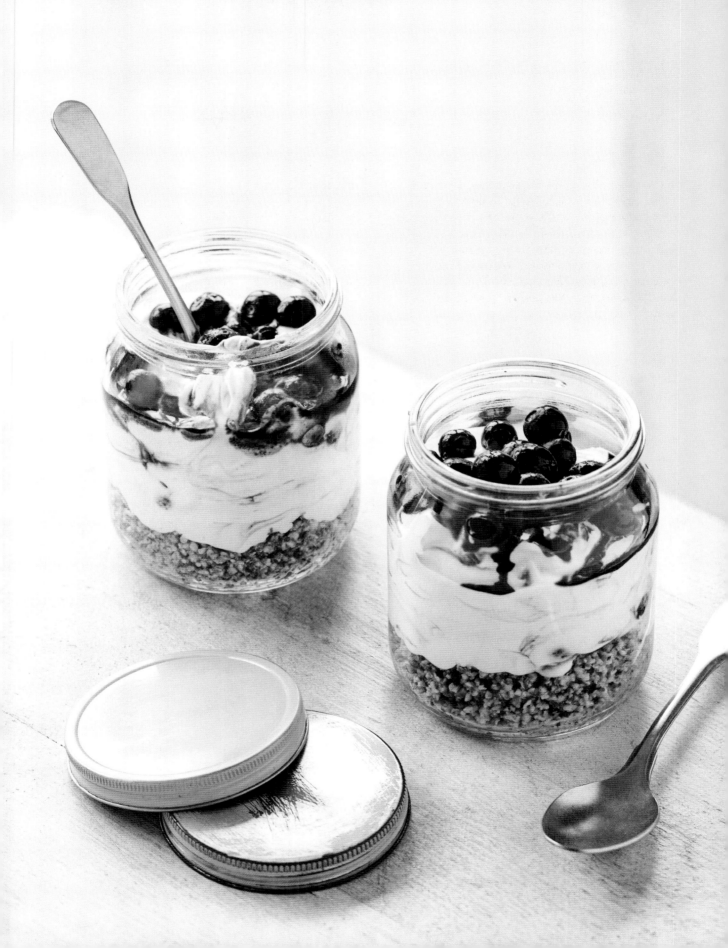

AZTEC HOT CHOCOLATE

MAKES 4 SMALL CUPS

This is a short, dark, rich hot chocolate shot rather than a big milky mugful. Similar to an espresso, it packs a powerful punch and makes a really warming treat after a winter workout or race. Dark chocolate with a high cocoa content has lots of nutritional benefits such as improving circulation, reducing 'bad' cholesterol and protecting skin and eyes, so you can happily indulge in this without any guilt!

100g dark chocolate
    (at least 70% cocoa solids), grated
1 tsp vanilla extract
Pinch of freshly grated nutmeg
½ tsp chilli powder (optional)
1–2 tbsp runny honey or maple syrup, to taste
2 cinnamon sticks, halved

1. Heat 500ml of water in a small pan until hot but not boiling. Add the chocolate and whisk over a medium-low heat until well combined and thick.

2. Stir in the vanilla extract, nutmeg and chilli powder, if using, then sweeten to taste with the honey or maple syrup.

3. Gently heat for a further 5–8 minutes, to allow the flavours to infuse. Whisk occasionally and be careful not to let the mixture boil.

4. Serve in espresso cups or small glasses with half a cinnamon stick to flavour and stir.

PER SERVING	
KCAL	165
FAT (g)	11.0
SATURATES (g)	6.0
CARBS (g)	13.0
SUGARS (g)	10.0
FIBRE (g)	3.0
PROTEIN (g)	2.0
SALT (g)	0.05

INDEX

D

ACKNOWLEDGEMENTS

Putting a cookbook together is a bit like running a marathon relay race – many talented people hold the baton at different stages and each of them, in turn, helps the project to cross the finishing line. I therefore need to say thank you to all the great runners in my team ...

Thank you so much to the amazing folk at Hodder & Stoughton for their vision, commitment and encouragement throughout: editorial director Nicky Ross, project editor Natalie Bradley, art director Alasdair Oliver, production manager Claudette Morris, marketing manager Catriona Horne and publicity director Louise Swannell. It's a dream team!

I am also very lucky to be supported by a great line-up behind the scenes. Many thanks to Camilla Stoddart and Annie Lee for their help with the words and to Anna Horsburgh and Rob Allison for their help with the food. An extra special thank you must go to nutritionist Kerry Torrens, who kept us all on track with a firm and patient hand – her knowledge and passion for her subject is hugely inspiring and she's a pleasure to work with.

The stunning pictures in the book are thanks to the winning combination of art director James Edgar, photographer Jamie Orlando Smith, food stylist Phil Mundy and props stylist Olivia Wardle. Thank you all.

Thanks also to the mighty Justin Mandel in the States and Rachel Ferguson in the UK for organizing my busy life and making sure I am where I am supposed to be every day. I couldn't make the distance without you.

I am also ever grateful to all of my trainers and the fellow cycle enthusiasts and tri-athletes that I've met who keep me pushing every day.

And lastly, thank you to my incredible family, who keep me going at the 25th mile and always inspire me to give my best. Tana, Megan, Jack, Holly and Tilly – you are my favourite training partners and the motivation for everything I do.

METRIC/IMPERIAL CONVERSION CHART

ALL EQUIVALENTS ARE ROUNDED, FOR PRACTICAL CONVENIENCE.

WEIGHT

25g	1 oz
50g	2 oz
100g	3½ oz
150g	5 oz
200g	7 oz
250g	9 oz
300g	10 oz
400g	14 oz
500g	1 lb 2 oz
1 kg	2¼ lb

VOLUME (LIQUIDS)

5ml		1 tsp
15ml		1 tbsp
30ml	1 fl oz	⅛ cup
60ml	2 fl oz	¼ cup
75ml		⅓ cup
120ml	4 fl oz	½ cup
150ml	5 fl oz	⅔ cup
175ml		¾ cup
250ml	8 fl oz	1 cup
1 litre	1 quart	4 cups

VOLUME (DRY INGREDIENTS – AN APPROXIMATE GUIDE)

Rolled oats	1 cup = 100g
Fine powders (e.g. flour)	1 cup = 125g
Nuts (e.g. almonds)	1 cup = 125g
Seeds (e.g. chia)	1 cup = 160g
Dried legumes (large, e.g. chickpeas)	1 cup = 170g
Grains, granular goods and small dried legumes (e.g. rice, quinoa, sugar, lentils)	1 cup = 200g

LENGTH

1cm	½ inch
2.5cm	1 inch
20cm	8 inches
25cm	10 inches
30cm	12 inches

OVEN TEMPERATURES

Celsius	Fahrenheit
140	275
150	300
160	325
180	350
190	375
200	400
220	425
230	450